$15

The Mindful Way
Drug Addiction Recovery

Christopher Dines is a British mindfulness teacher and writer. Christopher came into recovery from drug addiction in 2004. He has published seven books and facilitated workshops, seminars, retreats, school talks and corporate events, assisting people to reduce stress and enhance their emotional well-being and serenity.

D1050247

Mindfulness titles available from Sheldon Press:

Alcohol Recovery
Catherine G. Lucas

Anxiety and Depression
Dr Cheryl Rezek

Compassion
Caroline Latham

Keeping a Journal
Philip Cowell

Life Crisis
Catherine G. Lucas

Mood Swings
Caroline Mitchell

Pain Management
Dr Cheryl Rezek

Quit Smoking
Dr Cheryl Rezek

Stress
Philip Cowell and Lorraine Millard

A full list of titles is available from Sheldon Press, 36 Causton Street, London SW1P 4ST and on our website at www.sheldonpress.co.uk

The Mindful Way

Drug Addiction Recovery

CHRISTOPHER DINES

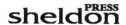

First published in Great Britain in 2019

Sheldon Press
36 Causton Street
London SW1P 4ST
www.sheldonpress.co.uk

British Library Cataloguing-in-Publication Data
A catalogue record for this book is available from the British Library

ISBN 978-1-84709-494-0
eBook ISBN 978-1-84709-495-7

Typeset by Fakenham Prepress Solutions
First printed in Great Britain by Ashford Colour Press
Subsequently digitally reprinted in Great Britain

eBook by Fakenham Prepress Solutions

Produced on paper from sustainable forests

To my late paternal grandma, Joyce Dines

Contents

Foreword

At least occasionally in the lives of us all, we experience tough times, whether it's loss of a loved one or falling prey to a terrible addiction that makes us feel hopeless and worthless. In *Drug Addiction Recovery*, Christopher Dines elegantly teaches us a process for healing from paralysing grief, addiction and emotional wounds using a mindfulness-based approach. He tells us that simply taking a step back to be the 'witness', while observing (but not identifying with) your thoughts, feelings and instinctive urges, will allow you to experience a greater degree of integration and balance in mind, body and brain. The key is to not have any one of your brain functions – be it instinct, emotion or intellect – dominate your life. When your instinctive urges, emotions and intellectual reasoning are harmoniously linked, recovery from addiction is possible. As Christopher tells us, this can happen when we step back to observe the instinctive feelings, thoughts and sensations the brain is bringing us. My good friend and co-author Dr Deepak Chopra taught complementary lessons in our books, *Super Brain* (Rider, 2013) and *The Healing Self* (Rider, 2018).

Instinctive urges are derived from the brainstem, which is responsible for the fight or flight responses, finding food and sexual drive. The brainstem and associated brain regions also ensure that you keep breathing, have a heartbeat and digest your food. In evolutionary terms, this is the oldest part of the brain, which is over three hundred million years old. Two hundred million years later, the limbic system in the middle part of the brain emerged. While the brainstem brings us programmed memories, our instincts (like finding our mother's breast for food as soon as we are born) and the limbic system brought us our first individual memories. Memories of what we found pleasurable led to our desires, while memories of what we found painful led to our fears. These were the first vestiges of acquired memories and they are tightly tied to emotions. That is why so many can remember in such amazing detail everything they did during the morning of the tragic events of September 11, 2001. Emotions and short-term memory are also handled by the limbic area in the mid-brain.

The newest part of the brain (which is only four million years old) is the prefrontal cortex, situated just behind your forehead. This is the centre of reason, meaning, purpose, creativity, empathy and self-awareness. It is also the area of the brain that allows you to step back and observe the base instincts, emotions and thoughts that are constantly creeping up and trying to dominate your attention. Simply put, the prefrontal cortex keeps our desires from becoming addictions, our fears from growing into unbridled phobias and our thoughts from becoming obsessions. This is the area of the brain that provides us with a sense of self, allowing us to be mindful, as opposed to being propelled by compulsive and impulsive behaviour.

This basic understanding of the brain is very important for people who suffer from an addictive behaviour, because addiction of all kinds makes us prone to compulsive and impulsive behaviour. To heal your emotional wounds, to shift from survival mode to one of thriving, Christopher Dines teaches us it's imperative that you do not try to edit, filter or regulate your thoughts and emotions – no matter how distressing or painful they may be. Whether you are grieving or coming to terms with a trauma or great loss, you will learn that the key is to not try to control your feelings, but sit on the beautiful mountaintop of consciousness and simply observe without judging. When you approach your emotional pain this way you automatically bring about a balance between your instinctive brain and the higher areas of your emotional and intellectual brain. Attaining that balance, by simple observation of your instinctive brainstem activities, emotional limbic brain functions and the self-awareness and intellectual processes of your frontal lobes, will help you to heal and thrive. You may also find yourself becoming calmer, more intuitive and generally happier.

In the wonderful book you are about to read, Christopher Dines gives you step-by-step exercises that will help you to integrate your brain and ground yourself in your body through guided mindfulness meditations, artistic expression and emotional training. Together with the personal stories, this book will be your precious guide for recovery and enable a renaissance of your mind, body and spirit. Enjoy the journey!

Rudolph E. Tanzi, Professor of Neurology,
Harvard Medical School

Acknowledgements

Thank you so much Sheldon Press for publishing this book and Fiona Marshall, Michelle Clark, Amy Carothers, Steve Gove, Elizabeth Neep and Norah Myers for your hard work and professionalism. Many thanks to Rudolph E. Tanzi (whose work has had such a positive effect on so many worldwide) for writing the foreword and for your continued support. Thank you to James Alexander, the late John Bradshaw, Dr Barbara Mariposa, Edward M. Frazer, Jeremy Thomas, Jonathan Lang, Kelly McNelis, George Stubbs, Joe Grahame, Mark Hatter, Melissa G. Jones, Jamie McBride, Jacinta Stephenson, David French, Sarah Barberis, Jeremy McGahan, Bekah Theisen, Mark Hambrook, Daniel Farnham, Michael J. McEvoy and Roger G. Thank you Peter Kyle MP for endorsing this book. Thank you, finally, to my beautiful partner Mary for your continued encouragement, for believing in me many years ago and for looking over the early drafts of this book.

Introduction
My story from 10 to 21

Between the ages of 10 and 21, my thoughts were consumed with how to escape reality – how to mask my feelings of inadequacy, shame, guilt, fear, abandonment, rage and loneliness. I desperately needed drugs and alcohol to mask my pain. I gravely abused alcohol, marijuana, cocaine, speed (amphetamine) and MDMA (ecstasy), and I once inhaled heroin. I was promiscuous and became addicted to watching online pornography.

I started drinking alcohol at the age of 10. This induced an intense sense of relief. Although in the beginning I was only drinking half a can or so of light beer, my addiction progressed at an alarming rate. By the time I was settled in my first year of secondary school, I was drinking alcohol and smoking marijuana every weekend. I was 12 years old. By 13, I intuitively knew that I was addicted to mind- and mood-altering drugs.

At the age of 14, I found myself in hospital having my stomach pumped due to alcohol poisoning. Four years later, I woke up in a hospital bed for a second time, again due to alcohol poisoning. Once I started drinking alcohol, I had almost no power inside me to stop. I would drink continuously for days until I collapsed physically and mentally. On countless occasions, I told myself that I would 'control' how much I drank, only to fail utterly.

Aged 15, I first tried cocaine, which induced a feeling of invincibility. I clearly remember going to a nightclub in the West End of London and feeling that I could take on the burly six-foot-six doormen (I was five foot six and quite thin) as a result of snorting cocaine. I became hooked the first time I used cocaine.

Several months later, I experimented with ecstasy. Although the experience was very pleasant, by the time I tried it again the following weekend, the 'rush' felt weaker and, within a very short space of time, my tolerance had heightened to the point where I was chewing ecstasy tablets while watching football games on weeknights, washed down with ample quantities of beer and wine. In my case, the illness of drug addiction progressed extremely quickly and my tolerance levels were dangerous.

My addictive behaviour spiralled on my first trip to Thailand in February 2004. I stayed dry for two weeks, then I relapsed and went on a dangerous drinking and drugging spree that lasted for two more weeks. I had a breakdown on my final night in Thailand. At 3 a.m., I decided to take a shower with my clothes on. I sat on the floor for hours sobbing. I eventually invited my friends into the room and, when they arrived, they were concerned to see water pouring from the shower into the hallway. The local Thai women working in the hotel were utterly baffled, although luckily my generous friends smoothed things out with the hotel manager. I was very lucky to return to London in one piece.

During that summer of 2004, I hit rock bottom – any sense of denial around my alcoholism and drug addiction had been utterly smashed. I was still living at my parents' home at the time and had been continuously abusing drugs over a 48-hour period. I came home in the late morning, when everyone was at work, and fell to my knees in the kitchen crying out loud for help. It's my belief that on that day, I connected with my spiritual centre and the beginning of my recovery was kindled. The idea of staying clean and sober, one day at a time, became a more attractive prospect than to continue drinking/drugging myself to death. It was as though, for 11 years, I had been in a deep hypnotic trance, which convinced me that, regardless of the harm I was inflicting on myself and my loved ones, it was perfectly fine to continue abusing alcohol and drugs. Hitting bottom was the best thing that happened to me. It saved my life and set me on a new trajectory.

Alcohol and drug addiction are probably the most widely recognized addictions, simply because they affect people in the most dehumanizing way. But people can become addicted to a range of substances and behaviours, from food to pornography, compulsive spending to gambling. These addictions also have a devastating effect on the children, parents and extended family of the person afflicted by them. One of the primary symptoms alcoholics and drug addicts exhibit is that they literally have an abnormal physical reaction when they put a mind- and mood-altering substance into their body. More often than not, they cannot moderate their alcohol or drug use. Once they start on a drug or alcohol spree, there is no stopping them. To compound the problem, without some sort of recovery programme, they find it extremely difficult, if not impossible, to cope with life without their 'medication'. They obsess about drinking alcohol or using drugs and, when they finally yield and put the mind- or mood-altering substance into their body, they kick off the whole cycle again. What worked for me, and has worked for millions of recovering drug addicts, was to physically stop using drugs, one day at a time (total abstinence). Then and only then can the mental and emotional dimensions of the drug addict be repaired.

Addicts are often suffering from suppressed – or 'frozen' – grief and the two separate conditions often heighten each other. Healing one's major emotional wounds will not cure a drug addict from his or her abnormal bodily reaction. Similarly, recovering drug addicts will never be able to use their choice of drug (cocaine, ecstasy, heroin and so on) safely, even if their grief has been addressed. Healing major emotional wounds, however, will certainly give a recovering drug addict enormous emotional release and greater freedom, clarity, courage and self-compassion.

Using this book

In writing this book, I hope to help you, as a recovering addict, deal with frozen grief and achieve self-compassion. In addition to new research and exercises, the book is based on a survivor's perspective and experience in recovering from chronic shame, addictive behaviours and frozen grief. While this book does offer you some intellectual stimulus and scientific data, the exercises are designed to activate your awareness at a *feeling level*.

If you are in therapy for addictive behaviour, complex post-traumatic stress disorder (CPTSD) or frozen grief, this book will add value to your personal emotional recovery. It might, however, be worth asking your therapist or counsellor to read the book before you participate in any of the exercises. Most fair-minded therapists and counsellors are happy for their clients to make use of books on emotional health and mindfulness, but it is better to check with your therapist to ensure it is not at variance with his or her own course of action.

If you are in a recovery-based programme or twelve-step fellowship, the book can complement and enhance your recovery. Primarily, it will resonate with people who have suffered with a drug addiction or multiple addictions and unresolved grief and who are familiar with the twelve-step model. Family and friends coping with a drug addict will also gain value from this book.

I have observed many professionals in the addiction field who find it very hard to thoroughly grieve their own traumatic childhood experiences. Naturally, this diminishes the efficacy of the treatment programmes they offer because the energy they are channelling to their clients lacks clarity; there is a lack of authenticity. Professionals who come into this category can also gain value from *Drug Addiction Recovery* if they are willing to open up about what is really going on inside them.

A particularly effective way to gain maximum benefit from the book is to ask a fellow traveller in recovery to join you. A small recovery group can be effective too, so long as its members are non-shaming and committed to long-term emotional and spiritual well-being. If you wish to work through the book with your spouse or partner, that can also be effective, so long as both people in the relationship are familiar with some sort of recovery programme and/or have attended therapy or counselling sessions.

When using the book you will need a journal to write in, a pen, paints and a paint brush (maybe even coloured chalk and pens) and a recording device. Nothing more is required, apart from your willingness to do the exercises in the book to the best of your ability.

Finally, I have used a variety of pseudonyms for recovering drug addicts mentioned in this book. While I have changed the names, the stories are based on real-life cases.

A cautionary note for recovering drug addicts

The main focus of this book is on assisting you in your personal recovery, not on 'curing' you of addiction. It is true, however, that an addict of any kind is less likely to relapse once emotional health has been restored. Gaining a sufficient long-term foundation in total abstinence recovery must *always* come first. In other words, this book is designed to complement your recovery, not replace it. It is almost impossible to address emotional wounds if an addict is still using drugs. Keep in mind that it takes at least three years of continuous total abstinence for the mind and brain of a recovering alcoholic or drug addict to clear.

Furthermore, while I believe recovering drug addicts need to exercise total abstinence (for example, quitting using heroin or cocaine entirely), I am in no way advocating that addicts who happen to be bipolar, for example, should stop taking the medication prescribed to them by their doctor. I know of many recovering drug addicts who have stopped illegal drugs but still carefully use prescribed medication under the supervision of their GP. Recovering drug addicts with bipolar disorder, schizophrenia, clinical depression or other severe mental health conditions will need extra medical assistance.

1

Running away and seeking oblivion

Generally speaking, drug addicts are afraid of their emotions. Many have spent years avoiding uncomfortable feelings by finding all sorts of ways to suppress them – what we might call 'numbing out' (by means of alcohol, cigarettes, food, drugs, sex, controlling people, compulsively fantasizing and so on). Many drug addicts dismiss their emotions by declaring, 'I don't do "feelings",' while some admit to being terrified at the prospect of getting in touch with their pain and therefore revert to self-medication by acting out in a destructive addictive behaviour. Others feel the need to present a mask to the outside world that 'everything is OK'; showing any sign of vulnerability or emotional pain would be an admission of 'weakness' and, more importantly, would put the addict in touch with decades of stored emotional and psychological pain.

Over the years I have seen many decent people in recovery from addictive behaviour who find it extremely difficult to direct compassion and kindness inwards and allow themselves to process their grief and trauma.

It is quite common for an addict to be in therapy for many years, know the diagnosis of her emotional condition and intellectually understand the solution, but be unable to release the emotional shackles that trap her in survival mode. Such a person might even claim, 'I've made the journey from my head to my heart' and believe it to be true. The person intellectualizing emotional health, however, still *feels* that something is not quite right. At an emotional level, life becomes harder and more frustrating, save for fleeting moments of excitement that mask the underlying pain. Such individuals use their intellect to suppress and push down painful memories and emotions. By and large, their emotional life is unpredictable and holds them back from fully living an authentic reality, one that honours their true values, needs and wants. Why are so many of these brilliant men and women still reporting that they cannot shift their emotional wounds? Why do so many of them still feel utterly flawed after years of attending support groups and studying literature on emotional intelligence?

Why, in particular, did Bill Wilson, the co-founder of Alcoholics Anonymous, write an open letter to recovering alcoholics in a 1958 *Grapevine* magazine article entitled 'The next frontier: Emotional sobriety', suggesting that the AA twelve-step programme, unaided, cannot engender emotional sobriety?* He wrote:

> I kept asking myself, 'Why can't the Twelve Steps work to release depression?' By the hour, I stared at the St Francis Prayer . . . 'It's better to comfort than to be the comforted.' Here was the formula, all right. But why didn't it work? Suddenly I realized what the matter was. My basic flaw had always been dependence – almost absolute dependence – on people or circumstances to supply me with prestige, security and the like. Failing to get these things according to my perfectionist dreams and specifications, I had fought for them. And when defeat came, so did my depression.

While gathering information about emotional health might be helpful, it is not possible to intellectualize, compartmentalize or rationalize emotional and spiritual well-being. I, too, used to intellectualize recovery. It does not produce satisfactory results. Unless our original pain is addressed, genuine emotional well-being and emotional intelligence are virtually impossible to realize. This is a process that cannot be 'forced', but we can certainly slow our progress by neglecting to feel our feelings.

Original pain

All children born into functional families will experience some degree of trauma. For instance, an infant might find it extremely difficult while attending nursery for the first time. He might weep for hours at a time,

---

* In the twenty-first century 'emotional sobriety' would more commonly be referred to as 'emotional well-being' or 'emotional health'. However, the term emotional sobriety is still used in some of the older twelve-step fellowships.

every day for a week, before he feels comfortable in his new surroundings. If the infant has a loving and emotionally healthy family, the child will have his feelings validated without being shamed. If, however, the infant has shaming and violent parents, the infant may develop a grave trauma. When emotionally wounded children grow up and suppress their feelings through addiction and self-harm, it is only by revisiting their original pain and grieving sufficiently that true mental, emotional, physical and spiritual healing, rather than temporary relief, can be realized.

Work on our original (childhood or adolescent) pain involves going back to our childhood and grieving any losses that we were unable to have properly validated. For example, if a child was sexually abused by a family member at a very young age, she might not consciously remember this tragic event; however, the traumatic event will be stored in her body. The event will affect her for the rest of her life unless she grieves this pain. The event might have been so traumatic that she left her body (her mind numbed out the abuse), but the residue will be stored in the muscles of her body. The suppressed traumatic energy stored in her body might manifest in chronic shame attacks, PTSD, poor relationships or antisocial and dysfunctional relationships. If, however, she develops a non-shaming support network and processes her suppressed original pain, she can recover from her losses and release dysfunctional survival traits.

In the twenty-first century we have more awareness of addiction and dysfunctional family systems, and how they relate to the human brain and body. We know that we can consciously rewire our brains and heal our emotional wounds by feeling our feelings.

Drug addiction is an illness

Without intervention, treatment and long-term recovery, addiction and addictiveness make us progressively mentally and emotionally ill. In my view, as well as that of scores of medical professionals and therapists, drug addiction is a chronic brain illness. When I use the term 'drug addiction', I am including alcohol addiction. Alcohol is a powerful, addictive mind- and mood-altering drug that can have devastating effects on one's health. In reality, an alcoholic is a drug addict who simply uses alcohol rather than, say, crack cocaine.

A recovering drug addict will never be able to return to his or her drug of choice even if he or she has been clean for decades. The illness of addiction – the addictiveness – progresses even if an addict is totally abstinent. There is a saying in the twelve-step community that when an addict is attending a twelve-step meeting, his or her illness is outside doing press-ups, waiting for the addict to show signs of complacency.

An individual with Type 1 diabetes can live a normal life with the right dose of insulin and regular monitoring, notwithstanding the fact that he will have to live with the condition for the rest of his life. Similarly, a drug addict can live the rest of her remaining years totally abstinent and even heal deep emotional wounds, but she is still wired in such a way that, without continuing to work on her recovery, relapse is likely.

Many emotionally wounded people have addictive behaviour; however, addictive behaviour and emotional wounds are two separate conditions (although a person may suffer from both). Thankfully, we can heal our addiction. But the process of recovery is a lifelong journey of self-discovery, open-mindedness, spiritual development, self-kindness and service to others, one day a time.

Addiction is often described as losing control over addictive behaviour to the point where it becomes destructive. Regardless of the destructive addictive behaviour, unless an individual can learn to feel his or her feelings, there is a high likelihood that one addiction will be swapped for another. Even if a cocaine addict quits using cocaine and alcohol, there is a strong possibility, unless she has addressed her addictiveness, that she will pick up another severe addiction, such as some form of eating disorder, a shopping addiction or a sex addiction. If a gambling addict quits gambling, he might start to drink heavily. Addictiveness can be expressed in two ways: through substance addiction and process addiction. Substance addiction includes the consumption of alcohol, cocaine, marijuana, heroin, prescription drugs or nicotine and, increasingly, 'legal highs' (such as benzodiazepines, morphine and so on). Process addiction includes addictions to sex, compulsive debting (compulsively using unsecured debt and living beyond one's means) and eating disorders, for example.

I came to respect the power of addictiveness when I quit drinking alcohol and found that, although I was physically sober, I was still vulnerable to other addictions. When I quit using alcohol, I stopped smoking cigarettes, but then started smoking cigars. I could feel that I was trying to change the way I felt by smoking cigars and so I decided to quit smoking altogether. I have not smoked since then.

Four years sober from alcoholism, I felt suicidal and went into a new recovery programme to address my addiction to online pornography and my love avoidance. While grieving in early recovery, and coming to terms with the realization that I needed help to have a healthy relationship with a woman, I turned to food to find comfort and quickly put on weight. I found temporary relief in overeating. Whenever emotions were intense, I 'fixed' myself with food. This continued for about a year until I continued to grieve in recovery and began to heal emotionally and spiritually. This cycle of swapping one addiction for another forced me to recognize the power of untreated addictiveness.

Below are some of the behaviours often expressed by a person in the cycle of an addiction.

- Drug addicts are in denial about their addictive behaviour.
- Consequently they go into hiding and often isolate themselves from others to indulge in their addiction.
- There is secrecy and a lack of transparency around their addictive behaviour.
- Drug addicts will lie to those closest to them if and when they are confronted about their addiction.
- They might become rageful or very controlling if they feel that their addiction is under threat from an external source.
- They will justify and rationalize their behaviour even when 'caught out'.

And here are some of the patterns found in addictive behaviour.

- The drug addict will, for example, stop snorting cocaine and drinking alcohol.
- The addict will aquire a new addiction, such as bingeing on chocolate or junk food.
- The addict might have a moment of clarity, stop bingeing on food and start attending the gym compulsively every day to lose weight and get physically fit.
- The addict, now in good physical shape and feeling much more confident, starts to compulsively act out sexually.
- The addict stops being promiscuous and is now trying

to battle a credit card addiction and/or compulsive debting, while still carrying suppressed grief and pain.

In this way, the addict is still locked into addictiveness regardless of overcoming several previous addictive behaviours.

2

Emotional wounds

Accepting our emotional wounds

Elizabeth's story
At the age of 35, a woman named Elizabeth sought professional help
for her feelings of rage and her inability to have healthy, intimate
relationships with men. She was either promiscuous or completely
avoided any sexual contact. Elizabeth deeply distrusted men, but had
a compulsion to take care of her father. She also happened to be a
recovering cocaine addict and alcoholic (she was ten years clean).
Whenever she started to get close to someone, she felt terribly guilty
and believed that she was abandoning her father. She would subconsciously find a way to sabotage the new relationship. Elizabeth's
mother had divorced her father and moved to a different continent
when she was 21. Her father never remarried but had a string of girl-
friends and occasionally slept with sex workers.

One day, after a complete meltdown with a new boyfriend,
Elizabeth started to have flashbacks of her father beating and raping
her mother in the kitchen. Elizabeth was three years of age at the time
but had blocked this horrific memory for over 30 years. At first, she
dismissed the memory and carried on with her life for another nine
months. The memory became clearer, however, and visited her fre-
quently. Whenever it resurfaced, she broke out in sweats and started
to shake. Finally, when her denial around the incident diminished, she
sought professional help and realized that she had never grieved the
reality that she had been abandoned during her most vulnerable childhood moments and had lost something for ever.

Elizabeth started to reflect on her parents' marriage and grad-ually came out of denial. There had been a great deal of verbal and emotional abuse and often physical violence in her family home, the memory of which she had blocked out. When she shared her revela-tions in a support group, she came to understand that she was actually terrified of her father, which was why she could not commit to another man and settle down. Furthermore, she realized that she had carried the trauma with her and was a victim of emotional incest, as a result of witnessing her father rape her mother. Her sexuality was fractured and her coping mechanism had been to sexualize her suppressed emo-tional wounds by being promiscuous or, conversely, starving herself of any form of sexual and emotional nourishment.

When, however, Elizabeth went through her grief work (the work she underwent to heal her grief in order to enhance her recovery) and felt her emotions deeply without using any coping mechanisms to distract herself, her relationship with herself and others improved dramatically. She eventually married a man and was no longer terrified of her father. Her denial with regard to her emotional wounds had gone and she was able to work on being authentic for the rest of her life, one day at a time.

As in Elizabeth's case, a drug addict will have suppressed emotional pain that will need to be felt mindfully and validated at some point in recovery, otherwise the risk of a relapse is far greater. In this chapter, we will explore some of the dysfunctional thought patterns, limiting beliefs and emotional wounds that often heighten addic-tive behaviour. Once a drug addict is physically clean, the next step in the lifelong process of recovery is to make peace with the past, so that the addict can be present and live authentically.

It is much easier to acknowledge a physical wound and seek help for it than to recognize and uncover an emo-tional wound or buried hurt that we may have carried inside us for many years. We subconsciously know that to accept that we are carrying entrenched emotional pain will seriously shake up our reality and potentially challenge our entire outlook on life. Many of us are terrified of the prospect.

For example, if we have to face the fact that we were abused in childhood, the recovery process might appear to be utterly overwhelming. For many people, this is too much to face. They convince themselves that it is easier to carry on and hope for the best, while secretly feeling disgusted with themselves, like a fraud and an imposter. For many people, living in denial appears to be a much easier and less painful prospect than exposing, exploring and grieving their suppressed pain. Some of us are such good 'actors' that even when unexpected traumatic memories resurface in adulthood, we can still behave as if nothing had happened, even while interacting with those who abused us many years ago. We turn a blind eye, justify, rationalize and continue the dance of self-delusion.

Many people live an entire lifetime without processing their pain, while unconsciously using denial as a shock absorber. While denial can serve a purpose as a coping mechanism, particularly for children and young adults, there comes a time in adulthood when it becomes a liability rather than an essential survival trait. Furthermore, there can be a high price to pay for a life lived in denial. The person in this state must tirelessly burn energy by presenting a false self to the world: 'Look how tough I am', 'I don't trust anyone', 'I'm incredibly self-sufficient'. The example of Elizabeth reveals how denial in adulthood can become an unbearable burden.

Emotional rock bottom

Most people need to reach some sort of emotional rock bottom before they are willing to do their deep feeling work, let alone address an addiction. This is why, in my view, hitting rock bottom can be a springboard to an immeasurably better life. When we hit rock bottom with an addictive behaviour or in coming to terms with a traumatic childhood, we open ourselves up to new possibilities. We can address the problem with clarity. We can reach out for help and build a social recovery network. The hope is that a person can hit rock bottom with as little external damage as possible, although some people need a major crisis (or many crises simultaneously) before they can come to terms with the pain they have been running away from.

Deep feeling work

Deep feeling work is an important part of the process with regard to restoring one's wholeness and authentic self (the True Self). By feeling our feelings deeply instead of attempting to mitigate the reality of our emotional pain, we can allow recovery to occur. Deep feeling work can only be effective if practised in the present moment with a willingness to feel intense emotions of sadness, loss, anger, betrayal and so on. The writer and workshop speaker John Bradshaw regularly lectured and talked about the importance of deep feeling work in order to overcome 'the hole in the soul' and, therefore, addictive behaviour.

Emotional health can be restored when an addict comes out of denial about the pain he has repressed, as the denial can then be processed and validated. A good counsellor, therapist or mindfulness practitioner will be able to assist during this highly sensitive process, as will a non-shaming support group.

Childhood abuse

Childhood abuse (mental, emotional, physical, spiritual or sexual) is often the primary cause of our emotional wounds and can certainly heighten a grave addictive behaviour. When we practise our deep feeling work, memories of childhood abuse and disturbing flashbacks often appear. We might have developed emotional wounds due to neglect and abandonment. Childhood abuse can manifest in many ways:

- being regularly screamed at or assaulted;
- being mentally, emotionally, spiritually and/or sexually abused;
- being a victim of emotional incest;
- witnessing violence;

- being constantly condemned and criticized;
- being shamed in public;
- being denied essential material comforts;
- being used by emotionally wounded parents to fulfil their needs;
- having one's feelings rejected and not validated;
- being expected to be 'flawless' and 'perfect' in a rigid or authoritarian family system.

Attachment trauma

Dr Bruce D. Perry's work on attachment trauma has brought tremendous clarity about the impact of early trauma on a child's brain. More recent evidence has shown that, moreover, the brain of a child exposed to a severe trauma such as mental, emotional, sexual, physical, religious or verbal abuse begins to wire itself in a different way from the brain of a child who has been nurtured in an emotionally healthy home. In other words, when a child is exposed to constant abuse, its neurological and emotional development will be impaired and its spiritual health will be compromised. Furthermore, without sufficient recovery, the person suffering from attachment trauma will be affected for the rest of his or her life (though, thankfully, the impact can be reduced).

In its first four years of life, a child primarily operates from the non-dominant (emotional) hemisphere of the brain; in other words, at a feeling level of awareness. This is why, as I go on to explain in Chapter 3, talking therapy alone is insufficient to heal one's earliest child-hood wounds. It is only by getting in touch with those stored feelings that emotional and spiritual health can be restored.

Self-loathing

There are all sorts of ways that self-loathing can mani-fest as a result of childhood abuse. I have seen countless children over the years being screamed at and utterly humiliated by their parents in public. It is not uncommon to see parents shame their children on a train or in a shop. Even worse, it is still perfectly legal for a child to be bullied for so-called 'bad behaviour' without passers-by so much as batting an eyelid. All these humiliations can compound themselves and create a web of self-hatred and deep, seething resentment. I am not suggesting that all childhood abuse leads to drug addiction, because that is simply not the case. I am saying, however, that children with a family history of drug addiction are unfortunately much more prone to become full-blown drug addicts if childhood abuse also occurred.

I, too, hated myself until I stopped drinking and got sober. I hated myself for becoming hooked on alcohol and being a full-blown drug addict by the age of 13. I hated myself for not being able to stop taking drugs in my teenage years and for sabotaging opportunities to improve my life. I loathed myself for hanging around with people who had no boundaries and who could not be trusted. I honestly believed that I was 'stupid' and gravely and irreversibly damaged.

Self-loathing is progressive

Anyone who directs hatred at anyone else hates themselves as well. After all, they are carrying hatred in their system. A decision to hold on to such heavy and raw emotions is certainly not an act of self-kindness. Many of us do not know how to adequately address self-loathing and, because it is so overbearing and intense, we often direct it at other people. This can be very dangerous. We might become bigots, racists, sexists or flirt with antisocial, fanatical religious groups. Some people who carry self-hatred might join a dark cult or follow a political group that promotes ideological extremism.

Hatred is passed down, a process that is multigenerational. If two parents hate themselves and bring up a child in a dysfunctional and emotionally unstable environment, the child will absorb hatred and direct it inwards. The child has no choice! A child can only absorb what it is subjected to. The child might lash out and become violent or internalize the toxic emotions, creating a web of self-loathing. Additionally, if the child has an addictive personality he or she will probably seek to self-medicate or turn to self-harm.

Owning our hidden dark side

Carl Jung believed that every person has a shadow that contains the darker elements of human nature. Seemingly intelligent people can express hatred, violence, selfishness, jealousy, spite or sadism. As you reveal your human shadow, you might feel ashamed or guilty about some of the perverse thoughts that fester in your mind. You might be terribly embarrassed to admit that you dislike people from different countries. You might find that you resent the opposite or the same sex. Many racists and sexists build images and ideas about an entire group of people that are founded on incomplete stereotypes and poor information. They learn to dehumanize the group of people they resent, which creates deeper layers of hatred in their minds. The good news is that as you come to own your shadow, it no longer has any power over you.

Age regression

Often when drug addicts are confronted with conflict or find themselves in an argument with their spouse or another family member, age regression manifests itself. For instance, a fully grown, mature man might be triggered by an event or by a person and, consequently, regress emotionally and act like a distraught six-year-old boy. When an unhealed emotional wound is prodded by a sarcastic comment, a smell or even a facial expression, old survival traits can appear and take over. A woman might stop thinking rationally and revert to behaving like a terrified and confused girl.

This can be very distressing for the person who has regressed. It is almost as though the individual travels back in time to the past and relives a moment when she was confused as a child, unable to have her pain validated.

If two emotionally wounded addicts in a relationship are triggered in this way and both regress to a time when they were abused in childhood or adolescence, things can get very ugly indeed. During the earlier years of my relationship with my partner, I sometimes emotionally regressed into childish behaviour. Today, however, I can feel when my old survival traits emerge. I allow myself to feel the pain and know that something or someone has revealed an unhealed emotional wound.

PTSD and PTSS

Many people who identify as drug addicts can be diagnosed as having post-traumatic stress disorder (PTSD) as a result of being exposed to particularly traumatic events. In an interview with me for *The Huffington Post UK* (Dines, 2017), Claudia Black, a pioneer of the adult children of alcoholics movement, explains, 'PTSD is often described as a set of accumulated, chronic, unprocessed fight, flight and/or freeze responses'. Someone who has been raped or sexually abused, has fought in a war or been continually and severely beaten is more likely to suffer from PTSD than someone who has not been subjected to physical violation (although this is not an absolute). According to Dr Shamini Jain (Jain and Chopra, 2015), 'One grave traumatic event in childhood is as serious as three years in a combat zone.'

While most addicts have trauma trapped in their bodies, it does not necessarily mean that they have PTSD. Some, however, may have post-traumatic stress symptoms (PTSS), as described by Claudia Black (Dines, 2017): 'The term post-traumatic stress symptoms is a newer term which describes the more common and less severe short-term trauma responses. And even more will experience consequences more subtle but nonetheless hurtful to their lives.'

Survivor's guilt is one symptom of PTSD. Someone with survivor's guilt feels that by surviving a deeply distressing and traumatic event they have done something wrong. The term survivor's guilt was recognized in the 1960s by therapists who were working with Holocaust survivors.

Complex PTSD

Research by Harvard's Dr Judith Herman has brought much more clarity with regard to complex traumatic issues, expanding on PTSD. For example, people who have been subject to continuous psychological, emotional, sexual or physical violence (or all of them combined) may be suffering from complex PTSD. Drug addicts, the adult children of alcoholics or drug addicts and violent families are often diagnosed as having CPTSD. Long-term domestic violence, child abuse of whatever kind, growing up in a grave drug-addicted, dysfunctional family and so forth are all traumas often associated with CPTSD.

Hypervigilance

Hypervigilance can often be a symptom of PTSD and associated disorders. If a boy has been subjected to the rage of a father who regularly smashed up the home and, consequently, absorbed years of trapped trauma stored inside his body, he will be on 'high alert' most of the time. He will feel intensely anxious, uptight and pumped up with adrenalin. He will frantically scan his environment to see if it is safe.

For example, a man named Jacob reported that, as a boy, he grew accustomed to his parents coming home from work and fighting with each other almost every evening. They hurled vitriol at each other for up to an hour and occasionally became physically violent. Cutlery, lamps and drawers were often smashed and broken. Whenever Jacob heard his parents' car pull up in the driveway, he panicked and would instantly relive the trauma of witnessing his parents fighting with each other.

Similarly, a woman named Briony said that as a girl she spent a lot of energy looking out of her front room window because she wanted to know in advance if her father was about to unlock the front door and enter the house. She wanted to avoid seeing him. As a result of this, whenever she heard a key turn in the front door, she relived trapped trauma in her body. Consequently, Briony became hypervigilant as an adult. She compulsively assessed people's facial expressions, scanned her environment for potential conflict, looked behind her while walking and monitored the body language of almost every person walking past her apartment 'just in case'. If she was too overwhelmed, she would compulsively clean her home to distract her from her pain.

The wounds of generational drug addiction

A family is a social system and if that system is dysfunctional, the ramifications for the children growing up within it are grave. In what is known as generational drug addiction, the adult children of drug addicts and alcoholics are quietly suffering all over the world. By the time the children have grown up, dysfunction has been deeply ingrained in mind, body and brain. The adult children of drug addicts become co-dependent and often exhibit various addictive behaviours. Addictiveness and dysfunction trickle down through the generations.

Common unspoken rules in dysfunctional families are: *do not, under any circumstances, talk about what is really going on for you and don't talk about the family's dysfunction to outsiders; don't talk about your true feelings; don't trust yourself and don't trust anyone else; don't feel your feelings; deny your feelings and suppress them by any means.*

If a child's parent is a drug addict, it is impossible for the dysfunctional parent to be fully emotionally present for that child. If a drug-addicted parent views himself as 'defective' or 'flawed', the emotional toxicity and trapped frozen energy must be fully absorbed by the child. Untreated drug addicts who try to heal their own emotional pain by having children can only pass on their suffering to their children.

Some addicts try to live their unfulfilled dreams through their children. Others simply use their children as an emotional fix to soothe their loneliness and heal their own childhood trauma. If a parent had her own needs neglected as a child, she will be triggered when the child is asking for attention. When dysfunctional parents realize that their children cannot fix them any more, they will either wish to be rid of their children or seek to control them for as long as possible (unless the drug-addicted parents are able to get clean and grieve their losses).

Adult children of a drug addict believe that they are responsible for their parents' well-being. If her parents are unhappy, the adult child feels that it is her fault. If his parents are angry, the adult child feels that he caused it. The adult child feels that she has to please her parents and 'smooth out arguments' in the family – to be an emotional shock absorber. She cannot fathom that she is utterly powerless over the dysfunctional behaviour of her parent or family of origin. The fact is that it is neither the child's nor the adult's job to try and shape the way her parents see the world, nor is it her responsibility to fix them.

The adult child, regardless of his own achievement or lack of it, cannot be free and content without going back to his childhood and grieving his losses. The adult child of a drug addict will always feel that something is missing in his life. Such adults will feel hollow inside, regardless of whether they are married and have children themselves. If they are personally rejected in the slightest way, they feel unloved and abandoned.

Family enmeshment and triangulation

There is a difference between healthy bonding and what is known as 'enmeshment'. Healthy bonding occurs when two people can be intimate and authentic with each other and have an understanding of both parties' humanness. No one is playing out a dysfunctional family role; there is a mutual respect for each other's boundaries and personal sense of self.

In dysfunctional families, however, boundaries are very unclear or virtually non-existent. A parent will often disclose inappropriate information to his or her child. Siblings have a chronic sense of entitlement towards each other. Family members will often take it upon themselves to fix and control other members' affairs and turn nasty or play the victim when they are confronted for fixing and controlling. Being autonomous and having the right to separate as an individual from a dysfunctional family is unacceptable when family members are enmeshed within the family social system. False loyalty and toxic guilt are common emotional weapons that are used when someone attempts to become an individual and no longer wishes to be responsible for other family members' feelings and behaviours. By and large, there is no respect for an individual in an enmeshed and dysfunctional family. In a system of dysfunctional family roles identified by author and counsellor Sharon Wegscheider, the individual is used as a piece of a puzzle to fit into a family role: hero, scapegoat, martyr, mascot, forgotten adult child.

An example of enmeshment is when Lauren (an older sibling) arranges to meet Jessica (her younger sibling) for lunch in a restaurant. Jessica then invites her parents without asking Lauren if this would be acceptable. She does so in order to extract money from them and the parents go along with it in an attempt to control and influence their offspring. Lauren turns up and finds out that Jessica has invited their parents without asking her. Lauren feels angry because she wanted to avoid seeing her parents for a few weeks, as a result of the parents behaving in a very toxic way the previous week. Therefore, she confronts Jessica, which leads to an argument in the restaurant. The parents arrive in the middle of the argument and intervene by shaming both siblings. Lauren feels unheard, Jessica feels confused and the parents feel superior. All four members of the family are enmeshed.

Rigid control versus harmonious order

Generally speaking, drug addicts are obsessed with control. They will go to extreme lengths to attempt to control outcomes, circumstances and other people's thoughts, feelings and actions. They are themselves subject to rigid control. This illusion of control might have been a necessary defence mechanism in childhood, as a result of growing up in a chaotic and frantic home. Nonetheless, the compulsion to control stifles one's creativity and joy.

Most addictive families are governed by rigid control. This can be expressed through a totalitarian family system where one parent or guardian is a frightening authority figure. All in all, members of an addictive family are obsessed with manipulating their fellow members' emotions.

Rigid control can manifest in the following ways:

- obsessing about how to control other people's behaviour;
- going to great lengths to control how people think and feel;
- resenting people who resist one's rigid control;
- exhibiting a lack of spontaneity and the need to rigidly stick to plans;

- a compulsion to control one's own thoughts and feelings instead of simply observing them.

In contrast, when we let go of rigid control, harmonious order can manifest in ways like these:

- being OK when we have to suddenly adjust or change our plans;
- feeling the urge to do something spontaneous and creative on a regular basis;
- not having a compulsion to control outcomes – being able to let go and appreciate the present moment;
- keeping a focus on improving one's own shortcomings instead of trying to fix other people's faults;
- having a curiosity about different subjects;
- a growing desire to explore and travel – to experience new cultures and perhaps learn a new language, musical instrument or about a new subject;
- letting go of pettiness;
- rekindling a desire to participate in and/or explore artistry;
- having a healthy desire to contribute to the greater good in one's own authentic way.

Depression

Most drug addicts have a history of depression. During my active alcohol and drug addiction, I would probably have been diagnosed as being clinically depressed. In recovery, I still suffer from mild depression, which comes and goes. Thankfully, my recovery and mindfulness practices have seriously dented the effects of this condition.

There are different types of depression such as mild depression, bipolar, clinical depression, post-natal depression and seasonal affective disorder (SAD). A person will require medical assistance to deal with their depression, typically if diagnosed as being clinically depressed or bipolar.

Hopelessness

Prior to coming into recovery, addicts often silently live in a state of chronic hopelessness. By and large, such a state manifests as a result of years of back-to-back disappointments and suppressed grief or untreated addiction. Hopelessness prevents us from revealing our own inner light and the talents we have to offer the world. Hopelessness convinces us that no matter what we attempt to do, we will always fail and therefore confirm our uselessness to ourselves and others. The paradox is that when we admit we feel hopeless, we can start to talk about what is really going on inside and therefore be in a position to receive help. Hopelessness can be replaced with hope when we talk about our losses and disappointments with people who can personally show empathy. Self-compassion can dissolve a sense of hopelessness.

Compare and despair

While being inspired by other people can rejuvenate one's mental and emotional well-being, compulsively comparing oneself to others can be destructive and frustrating. Addicts often compare themselves unfavourably to others and, consequently, dissatisfaction and rage regularly hijack their emotional state. Often an addict will compare his experience to a snapshot of someone else's life on social media or in a magazine, giving himself another wonderful excuse to direct debilitating criticism inwards. Thus the saying 'Compare and despair'.

Toxic shame and guilt

The late John Bradshaw used to write and lecture on what he termed 'toxic shame' and its debilitating effects. He was able to communicate ever so elegantly that 'moral shame' (guilt) was needed in order to develop a positive moral compass, but conversely 'toxic shame' caused an addict to feel utterly flawed. In the foreword to my book, *The Kindness Habit* (2016), Bradshaw shared the following views:

> Addictiveness is rooted in toxic shame. Shame is a natural affect. It exists to help us form our early sense of identity; it guides us to form a conscience and a sense of guilt (moral shame). Without the effect of shame, the foundation of our moral life would collapse. As the philosopher Nietzsche said long ago, 'Everybody needs a sense of shame, but nobody needs to be ashamed.'

Toxic shame caused me a great deal of suffering in the first 21 years of my life. It gravely dented my self-worth, self-esteem, dignity, personal and professional relationships and finances and prevented me from being authentic. Unhealed chronic, toxic shame wrecked countless opportunities to expand my professional life and therefore caused me to be plagued with the fear of financial insecurity.

I have realized from my own experience, and from listening to my fellow travellers in recovery, that sometimes guilt can be as toxic as chronic shame. For example, many emotionally wounded addicts feel guilty when they speak out and stand up for themselves. They feel guilty for putting their own well-being first or for saying 'No' to someone. That is not healthy guilt.

Shame attacks

Shame attacks are a symptom of toxic shame that is stored inside the human body. An addict can walk into a restaurant and suddenly have a gut-wrenching emotion rushing throughout the body – feelings such as 'I'm ugly . . . disgusting . . . flawed . . . unlovable . . . a fraud . . . less than'. Shame attacks can be triggered by the most unremarkable events. We might smell a scent that subconsciously reminds the body of a shameful or traumatic event. We might walk past someone who resembles a person who shamed us.

Shame attacks can be reduced if we are able to feel the emotions underneath them. Even when shame attacks come to the surface after we have processed our grief, shame is greatly diminished. We can say to ourselves, 'I know this feeling. I am having a shame attack and it will pass.'

Voice shame and digital screen shame

Similar to shame-based people being subject to shame attacks when looking at themselves in the mirror, voice shame can be just as powerful. Often a shame-based person will loathe the sound of her own voice. She finds it excruciating to hear her voice played back to her on a digital family video or recording. Some shame-based people have found it very difficult to record their own voice for the purpose of participating in a scripted recovery meditation. Generally speaking, this chronic self-loathing stems from being mocked and teased during one's most sensitive and formative years. Voice shame can be overcome with self-acceptance and regular affirmations. It is essentially the unkind mental commentary about how we sound that is the problem, rather than the voice itself.

Shame-based people can also feel self-disgust when looking at themselves in a homemade video, such as one made of themselves for a video blog or a video diary they have recorded on their mobile phone. The critical inner voices can be incredibly harsh with respect to digital screen shame.

Anger, resentment and rage

Anger that is expressed in a healthy and civil way can be liberating. Anger is often produced to protect us so that we can assert a boundary. By and large, when we are angry, fear is the cause. We may feel angry if we are afraid that something will be taken away from us or that we will not get something that we want. We may feel angry if we are afraid that someone we love is being bullied or hurt. We may feel angry when we are afraid that we are being used or mistreated. This is natural. Learning to express our anger in an emotionally intelligent way is much healthier than suppressing it. Anger that is suppressed can harm the human body and cause depression. In recovery, we can learn to tell someone we are angry without raising our voices or screaming at them.

When we allow anger to fester inside us, however, it can lead to resentment, especially if we feel powerless to affect a situation. If a person is being abused or bullied by someone and feels powerless to do anything, the anger that person is feeling may transmute into resentment. Resentments quickly compound and replay themselves over and over again. Resentments are poisonous and diminish our mental, emotional and spiritual well-being. Resentments can lead to violence, revenge, hostility and animosity towards others – and more importantly towards ourselves.

Some of the stored resentment we carry is not our original resentment. Many people inherit resentment passed down by their parents or grandparents. They are carrying other people's feelings even though the animosity is not a consequence of their own personal experience.

Rage is static raw anger and resentment entrenched in the human body that can shoot through the entire system like a bolt of electricity. Inner rage is an explosive energy that lies dormant inside, but which when released can drive people to extreme acts of physical and emotional violence. Inner rage, like a shame attack, can be triggered by the most seemingly unremarkable events. A relatively harmless comment or the expression on someone's face can trigger a volcanic reaction in our bodies.*

Unless someone has done their major grief and original pain work, they will find it almost impossible to calmly handle inner rage when it flares up. Many addicts who have healed their serious emotional wounds have reported that doing physical exercise, such as pumping weights, power walking, jogging, yoga, punching a boxing bag or tai chi, have released the charge of static energy. Accompanied with deep breathing, this can be very helpful too.

---

* I became so fascinated with the concept of inner rage and how it once used to regularly affect me that I dedicated an entire chapter to it in my book, *Manifest Your Bliss: A spiritual guide to inner peace* (2013).

Emotional wounds self-appraisal

After you have read this chapter, I recommend putting some time aside to answer the questions below. It is important to gain as much clarity as possible about the issues hampering your mental, emotional and spiritual well-being. Answering the questions might bring up some emotional pain and discomfort. There is no need to rush when reflecting and answering them. If your feelings are too overwhelming, just stop writing. If you answer yes to more than two questions, it might be worth seeking help from a trained therapist, counsellor or mindfulness practitioner, as well as joining a weekly support group (a twelve-step meeting, for example).

1 Do you feel that you carry suppressed emotional wounds?
2 Do you believe that you have hit some sort of emotional rock bottom? If so, are you willing to do whatever it takes to heal?
3 Can you relate to childhood abuse? Were you consistently mentally, emotionally and/or physically abused as a child?
4 Were you subject to a cult-like religion that suffocated your personal spirituality? If so, what steps have you taken so far to heal these wounds?
5 As a child, were you a victim of incest and/or were you sexually abused in childhood or as an adolescent?

If so, have you discussed this with a safe confidant? Do you carry toxic shame and embarrassment with respect to incest? Is incest still a problem in your family of origin?

6 Do you have a tendency to defend people who are abusive and/or who have abused you?

7 Do you secretly loathe yourself? Do you feel fundamentally flawed and unlovable? Are you aware that self-hatred is progressive and deepens without thorough childhood grief work?

8 Are you aware of your dark 'hidden' side? For example, are you a silent racist or sexist, intolerant of 'foreigners' or people who practise a different religion from you?

9 Do you hate parts of your body? Are you unable to accept the colour of your skin or the 'imperfect' parts of your body?

10 Do you have a negative frame of mind most of the time? Are you constantly condemning yourself and others? Do you often feel jealousy or secretly wish harm on others?

11 Are you a shame-based person? Do you suffer from toxic guilt? Are shame attacks a problem for you?

12 Do you currently resent someone or a group of people? Are you often filled with explosive rage?

13 Have you experienced a grave trauma? Is trauma a problem for you?

14 Are you hypervigilant? Are you always looking out

for a potential threat even in the midst of safe and pleasant company?

15 Are you addicted to trying to control people, events and outcomes? Is rigid control something that you cannot shift?

16 Does your family of origin show signs of enmeshment and triangulation? Are you enmeshed with someone?

17 Do you recognize age regression in your behaviour when you feel threatened or confronted by a person and/or group of people?

18 Do you often feel depressed or despondent towards life?

19 Do you regularly compare yourself to others in a destructive way?

20 Do you loathe the sound of your own voice or seeing yourself on screen?

3

Processing frozen grief

Frozen grief occurs when we deliberately numb out and refuse to process our major losses. Frozen grief is essentially suppressed emotional pain (loss and abandonment) stored in the human body. Frozen grief torments drug addicts. Deep below the emotional surface of the drug addict who has yet to find recovery lies untold, suppressed pain and loss. In my view, frozen grief can stifle an addict's chance of accessing inner peace and serenity. In this chapter, we will explore the process of grieving the past so that we can live fully in the present and minimize emotional triggers.

The importance of grieving regularly

It has been said that bereavement is a state of loss and grief is a response to loss. To grieve is a natural and healthy response to our losses. It is nature's way of letting us heal and open ourselves up to a new chapter in our lives. Grief can occur in all sorts of ways. We can find ourselves grieving the death of a family member or friend, the loss of a job or career or else moving away from our childhood home; we may even grieve during the transition of power in government. Anything that sincerely feels like a loss in our lives can cause a grief response. The problem for many addicts is that we have never learned how to grieve properly or we have moved heaven and earth to avoid our pain.

Life is a series of changes and losses and, unless we grieve each loss as it occurs in the present moment, the suppressed emotions will compound themselves until we find one day that we have lost touch with *feeling*. We become emotionally numb, dissociate and live in our heads, shut off from intimacy and authenticity. We become too dependent on the intellect and forget how to feel our emotions in the body.

While the experience of being human can bring joy, creativity, bliss, enthusiasm, peace and transcendental moments of ecstasy, it is inevitable that it will also bring sadness, trauma, injustice, disappointment and suffering. Grief allows this cycle of human emotion to flow through our bodies and be processed in a harmonious way. Carrying around static and frozen emotion weighs us down, robs us of playfulness and of the ability to live in the present moment. It is important to *feel* the losses we have avoided feeling for so long, so that we have a better chance of dealing with any new misfortunes and vicissitudes. We might find that we have buried a painful memory that creates a string of uncomfortable emotions.

We might realize we have neglected to grieve a relationship or have not allowed ourselves to weep for several years (some emotionally wounded people have not wept in decades).

Why are you afraid to grieve?

Understanding why we are afraid to grieve is a prelude to transforming our lives. Getting in touch with our deepest fears and airing them in a safe space can be incredibly liberating. We heal and progress when we expose our fears with a recovery action partner or mentor (often called a sponsor in a twelve-step fellowship) or with a trusted friend. A sense of inner freedom and clarity can be rekindled when we regularly shine the light on our fears and are able to discard them.

For many emotionally wounded addicts, the idea of grieving is a daunting prospect. To regularly grieve does require courage and a desire to heal – but rest assured; the resulting gains from these efforts are profound. Personally, I was terrified of coming to terms with my past and having to let go of fixed ideas about myself and the world. I was afraid of accepting my losses and having to move on with my life. The fact is, I never learned how to process my losses and have my pain validated in a functional and compassionate way.

Below are some questions that might bring you more clarity about your grief. It is best to share your answers with a friend in recovery – a recovery action partner – or a professional and see what unfolds. You might be inspired to thrash out new ideas to improve your life or you might begin a new course of action.

1 Why are you afraid to grieve?
2 What do you think is stopping you from grieving?
3 Why have you been suppressing your pain? For example, do you fear that the emotional pain of your losses will be overwhelming?
4 Do you believe that you will lose control if you get in touch with your losses?
5 What do you think will happen to you if you get in touch with your frozen pain?
6 Are your fears rational and can you imagine yourself transcending your fears?
7 Why are you afraid to feel your emotions?
8 Do you act out in the form of an addictive behaviour when you begin to feel lonely, isolated and abandoned?

What do you need to grieve over?

Now that you have more clarity about why you are afraid to grieve, you can identify what you need to grieve over.

Some people are seeking to come to terms with the reality that they never truly processed the loss of a parent or a close family member. Some realize that they need to grieve over the loss of not having non-abusive parents while growing up, while others realize that they have not grieved the loss of opportunities missed as a result of being powerless over an addictive behaviour (an alcoholic, for example, might be riddled with self-contempt, having created self-inflicted wounds). Discuss what you need to grieve over with your action partner or therapist and allow yourself to receive some gentle, non-shaming feedback. The questions below are designed to bring further clarity about your need to grieve.

1 What do you need to grieve over?
2 Did you sufficiently grieve over your childhood?
3 If you were subject to abuse in childhood, did you have your pain validated by a sober and compassionate adult?
4 Did you grieve over being betrayed in childhood and losing your sense of innocence?
5 Have you grieved over any pain inflicted in your teens?
6 Did you have a pet that died and, consequently, you refused to grieve over?
7 If your parents divorced or compulsively fought and abused each other, did you grieve over the loss of a safe and secure home?
8 Did you grieve over a death in the family or did you numb yourself out by indulging in addictive behaviour?
9 Have you grieved over the pain, loss and sorrow caused by your addictive behaviours?

10 Have you come to terms with the impact your addictions have had on your personal life and the effect on those closest to you?
11 Have you grieved over the unmanageability in certain areas of your life caused by your addictions?
12 Have you grieved over your major failures and mistakes?
13 Have you come to terms with some of your most cherished dreams not being fulfilled?
14 Have you grieved over the dysfunction and generational pain in your family?
15 If you were seriously abused (mentally, emotionally, physically, sexually or religiously), did you have this pain validated by someone else in a non-shaming way?
16 If you are in the later stages of your life, have you grieved over losing a younger body and physically ageing?

Grieving generational pain and ancient family suffering

Imagine how violent a typical family household was 500 years ago, at a time when women found guilty of petty treason, heresy or adultery were burned alive in public. This is just one example of how inhumane the collective consciousness was in England until the Treason Act of 1790 abolished such barbaric treatment. It takes many families (violent or not) to build a society and a nation and, while collective violence has decreased over the centuries, dysfunction has continued to trickle down through the generations. Domestic violence, alcoholism, drug addiction, mental illness, trauma, incest, racism and authoritarian family systems have all endured into the twenty-first century. If previous generations have experienced hardship, the trauma of poverty will affect future generations in one way or another. If previous generations were driven by immense political and economic power, this will also affect future generations.

In hindsight, I never properly grieved over my paternal grandmother's death. I was very close to her as a child and the impact her death had on me was immense. I went back into school the day after she died unexpectedly of a sudden heart attack and landed myself in a lot of trouble. At my grandmother's funeral, I suppressed my emotions and hardened myself to the occasion. I stood next to my grandfather and noticed that he did not shed a tear throughout the service, so I decided to do the same. I somehow managed to completely suppress the immense loss I was feeling. I made up my mind then that I was not going to feel the pain and therefore accept the loss of my grandmother, not realizing that my grandfather probably wept in private. He was six foot two, a member of the Second World War generation, which encouraged the maintenance of a stiff upper lip at all costs in the face of life's hardships. It would have been unthinkable for him to break down in public and weep.

When, in early recovery, I started to feel my suppressed painful emotions with respect to my grandmother's death and the terrifying years in secondary school, I started to feel less anxious and more secure within myself. I became less afraid of being abandoned. I finally allowed myself to cry and looked at old photos of the two of us playing in her home or on holiday on the south coast of England in the 1980s. During this early stage of recovery, I also grieved over other adults from my childhood; often figures I had placed on a pedestal, including a handful of school-teachers who had my best interests at heart. I grieved over childhood school friends I had moved away from.

When my paternal grandfather died in the mid-2000s, it was much easier to process because I was almost two years clean and sober. It was harder to neglect my feelings because I was no longer using alcohol to medicate them. I was able to attend his funeral and pay my respects to him in a functional way.

In my eleventh year in recovery I started to grieve my generational pain. This was much harder and more intense than the previous grief work I had done. For example, I came to realize that members from older generations of my family had died of drug addiction. That unspoken grief would have had an impact on me in some way. When I realized that there were dysfunctional traits in me from generations going back hundreds of years it was very humbling indeed. My Zen and yogi friends call this generational grieving process 'cleansing our karma'.

Validating our anger

During the process of grieving we need to give ourselves permission to be angry at those who have hurt us. Many people in recovery struggle in this respect. They come into recovery and declare, 'I forgive this person', but it is nothing more than an intellectual idea. They *think* they have forgiven someone because they have prayed for the strength to forgive or because they think that they ought to forgive, thereby stopping themselves from feeling the anger and hurt they are carrying. We cannot grieve properly unless we are able to get in touch with our anger and have our hurt sufficiently validated. Sharing our anger with a trusted friend, therapist or fellow traveller in recovery (someone who properly understands the grieving process) is invaluable.

Numbing out our feelings

When I reconnected with my authentic self, I started to reflect on what it meant to be a mixed-race (bi-racial/dual-heritage) human being. I had never really thought about the meaning of diversity until I came into recovery. As a result of being intoxicated on mood-altering substances, I had numbed out my feelings around my ethnic and cultural heritage.

Having been brought up with a white father and a black mother, I found that exploring their family roots was essential for me to gain clarity about my own original pain. As a baby, a child and an adolescent I had felt comfortable with my father's parents – especially my paternal grandmother – and his Anglo-Irish family of origin, who lived in London. My mother's relatives lived in Kenya and the United States of America, although we visited Africa on several occasions in my childhood and her relatives visited England regularly too. The secondary school I attended was multicultural and multiracial and gave me access to friends from different backgrounds. While I have golden brown skin and probably look more Indian or Brazilian than African, my worries and concerns are not that different from those of my fellow human beings who have a lighter or darker skin colour. When I stopped numbing out my feelings around my ethnicity and multicultural upbringing, my love and reverence for all people grew enormously.

By and large, numbing ourselves happens when we use substances or process addiction to deaden our feelings. We might spend ten hours compulsively watching a drama series to avoid feeling anger towards our spouse or lock ourselves away bingeing on ice-cream or coffee to escape our feelings of rejection. While constructive fantasy can be brilliant if we are undertaking creative projects, a person who regularly numbs out might use fantasy to block the hurt he or she feels towards others. Although I have never met anyone who does not ignore their feelings once in a while, too much numbing out blocks us from grieving our losses. When denying our feelings becomes our comfort zone, it can prevent us from living authentically.

A stiff upper lip

People who often talk about keeping a 'stiff upper lip' are choosing to suffer in silence, isolating themselves from others and destroying a chance to be authentic and sincere. I have spent time with many male recovering addicts who have healed as a result of talking about their emotional pain and depression. Some of them fought in the first and second wars in Iraq; they are physically hard men and are certainly not 'weak'.

An emotionally wounded person might have years of information in his brain with respect to the mind and human behaviour. If he thinks that all he needs to do in order to fix his own pain is to study emotional health, however, trouble arises. We cannot heal just by talking about our pain. While talking therapies can be a good start during the healing process, it is allowing ourselves to feel our rawest and most sensitive emotions in the body that brings deep healing. Hours of weeping at a time, sometimes on and off for an entire year, may be necessary to properly and sufficiently release frozen emotion from our system. Allowing ourselves to feel our feelings is one of the kindest things we can do for ourselves. It is a way to nurture the very core of our being.

People who pretend they have it together in the midst of immense suffering are ultimately making matters worse. In other words, emotionally wounded addicts who pretend to be 'tough' are actually operating from a state of fear. They are terrified of not being seen as being super-human and will display all sorts of artificial roles to push down their feelings. Contrary to what many people have been taught, it takes courage to admit that one is suffering mentally and emotionally and ask for help.

Sadness

Sadness is a healthy and natural human emotion, one that often comes and goes. Unfortunately, sadness has been labelled a negative feeling; the opposite of happiness and therefore an emotion to suppress and alter. Although sadness can be a feature of depression and grief, they are quite different. Often sadness can be misdiagnosed as depression and vice versa. Depression is a mental illness and warps our thinking and perception of reality, gradually stripping away any joy or fun from our lives. Sadness is its own unique human emotion that, when validated, can be cathartic and very healing. When we allow ourselves to feel sad we find it easier to be kind to ourselves and others. There is something sacred about sadness. The emotion reveals our humanness and can be a catalyst for humility and grace.

Weeping

As I have found, it can be very freeing to allow oneself to shed tears. In my recovery, weeping has been a very helpful way to get in touch with my true self. Weeping is cathartic and keeps the human spirit vibrant. Thankfully, attitudes to men weeping or 'welling up' in public are changing. In recent times, we have witnessed global football stars weeping after losing in the final of a major sporting event and a US president crying at a press conference.

Being 'heard' is a crucial part of the grief process

In Western mainstream society there is a tendency to encourage people to quickly move on after some sort of loss. Society tells us that we can 'think' our way out of grief. While it is certainly true that to compulsively dwell in the past can be counterproductive, it can be even more damaging to try and rationalize grief and force or rush the process of self-healing.

Often people who are working through deep feeling and grief recovery will need to repeat their painful stories out loud. Most emotionally wounded addicts feel that they have never been truly heard (how could they when they have hidden their darkest secrets for many years?) Self-compassion often takes a long time to realize in one's heart and spirit and, until such a wonderful thing happens, voicing one's hurt is necessary. For the first six months of my major frozen grief work, my recovery partner and I talked for at least two to three hours a week. It was very cathartic and spiritually nourishing.

Feeling our feelings in the human body

The most profound way to heal is to go deep within the human body. The mindfulness body scan meditation, for example, encourages the meditator to bring a gentle awareness of every feeling, sensation, tingle, physical ache, pain or suppressed emotional static energy in the body. The process is incredibly effective because emotions and trauma show up in the human body. We know that memories of emotions are stored in the muscles and that is why, when a traumatic memory revisits, our whole body feels it. If we are triggered by some trauma, the body informs us through the clenching of our fists, feeling tense or sweating profusely. To regularly anchor ourselves in the human body is a tremendous way to support the healing process of our suppressed grief and silent suffering. When we feel the body, this is where a breakthrough happens.

Grieving sexual and emotional incest

Unfortunately, incest is still quite common and is rife in families with a history of addiction. It is not unusual to hear of a daughter being subjected to incest on the part of her alcoholic father or grandfather, or of the adult child of an alcoholic practising incest with her own children. Many recovering drug addicts, sex and love addicts or love avoidants have been victims of incest.

Incest and sexual abuse also has to be validated and grieved if emotional health is to return and flourish.

The nature of incest and sexual abuse brings with it a profound sense of shame that often stops people from processing the abuse.

Incest can also manifest itself at an emotional level. For example, if a father makes inappropriate comments about his daughter's sexual attributes, this can be called emotional incest. Emotional incest can be just as degrading as sexual abuse or physical incest. It can take a long time for someone to accept that they have been exposed to sexual or emotional incest, as there is usually an air of denial around it.

Grieving toxic addictive relationships

Letting go of toxic relationships, whether that be disentangling from a co-dependent relationship or an abusive 20-year marriage, can trigger a profound sense of abandonment. If a fully grown adult is accustomed to regularly being financially bailed out by his parents or carers, the idea of being fully financially self-supporting and, therefore, changing the dynamics of the relationship, may be a daunting one. Coming to terms with no longer rescuing a spouse or a loved one who is in the grip of a grave addictive behaviour can be equally frightening. We may have to let go of someone we put on a pedestal or we fear and this can be incredibly difficult to do.

As we learn to enhance and develop our emotional health, we may find that our relationships change or cease to exist and this will cause grief. If we do disentangle ourselves from co-dependent relationships, it is important to process the feelings that surface and to honour our pain. This is the only way through. We can suppress our emotional pain all we wish, but, nonetheless, the static emotional energy will be lingering inside us.

Grieving our lost careers and missed opportunities

Many people can omit to grieve the loss of a career or a creative project, moving home or leaving their country of birth. The thing to remember is that life is movement and change is inevitable, so loss is impossible to avoid. Emotionally wounded addicts find it harder to grieve than people who were brought up in a safe and emotionally healthy family home. Loss to an addict feels like a personal attack and triggers pain from the original childhood abandonment or family enmeshment.

Listening to childhood music to activate frozen pain

When we are in the process of deep feeling work, listening to the music of our childhood or adolescence can be a very effective way to activate frozen grief in our body. For example, I was born in 1983 and so I researched every single top 40 pop track from 1982 to 2001. I made a note of the biggest pop and rock stars in the 1980s and early 1990s, such as Michael Jackson, Madonna, Nirvana, Sting and Elton John, and listened to their albums. Towards the end of my deep feeling grief work, I started to listen to my parents' favourite recording artists. I relentlessly went through the music of the 1960s and 1970s and remained open to seeing if any of the songs stirred up frozen emotions and memories.

If you start to listen to a song that brings back old memories and painful feelings, this might be a sign that you need to address the suffering associated with the song. Similarly, if you listen to a song and, all of a sudden, you feel like weeping, allow yourself to do so. You might end up playing the song several times or for an hour repeatedly as you weep. This process is highly therapeutic.

Watching films to trigger your memories

Watching old films to activate memories and emotions in the body can be very helpful too. For example, at Christmas in 2015, just before I started my deep feeling work, John Candy's films from the 1980s were showing on television and watching them helped me to unlock some frozen grief. Revisiting classic Disney films also revealed hidden childhood emotions. It is as though these films had freeze-framed my emotional state from that particular time. Similarly, the act of revisiting classic black-and-white Hollywood films reminded me of spending time with my paternal grandparents at their home in Pinner, London. When I revisited films from my childhood, waves of sad emotions came up to the surface.

Grieving the injustices of the world

While there are many wonderful things happening all over the world, it is important to put time aside to empathize and grieve when our fellow human beings go through a psychotic episode. Many people, for example, practise grief meditation, which is a highly effective way to heal.

I recall watching the news on TV just before I started my own deep feeling work. The journalist showed a short clip of a man running to rescue a terrified two-year-old boy who had narrowly escaped being bombed in a war-torn country. The man picked up the boy and put him in the back of a van with several distraught women and elderly people. Shortly before the man was about to drive the survivors to safety, another young boy no older than three years of age appeared out of nowhere and ran to the man, screaming for help. Thankfully, the man was able to save him from being left behind.

Two things happened to me. First, I was able to access my own lost inner child and, second, I felt compassion at a very deep level and wept profusely. It is essential to regularly grieve the injustices of the world – it develops humility and deep compassion in one's heart.

A grief inventory

Here is a list of questions that might help to bring more clarity to your grieving.

1 Do you feel that you properly grieved when your loved ones died? For example, a workaholic (before coming into recovery) might have numbed his or her feelings when a loved one died by working an excessive number of hours a day.

2 Did you sufficiently weep over the loss of loved ones?

3 Did you talk to anyone about your grief during the time of your loss?

4 Have you ever grieved over your childhood and adolescence?

5 Do you regularly well up and then push down your emotions to stop yourself from weeping?

6 Do you suppress your emotions when your body needs to release tears? If so, what do you feel that you are running away from?

7 Are you able to shed tears when you feel that you need to?

8 How often do you put time aside to sit with emotions of sadness and feel them unreservedly?

9 Do you feel that you are in denial with respect to your losses?

10 Have you sufficiently grieved being emotionally abandoned in your childhood?

4

Other addictive or dysfunctional behaviours

Drug addicts will likely suffer from other addictive or dysfunctional behaviours. Seldom will you meet a drug addict who does not exhibit multiple addictive behaviours. Because drug addiction and eating disorders are impossible to ignore so are often in the spotlight, often subtler addictive behaviours, such as love addiction, compulsive underearning and sex addictions, may be neglected. For this reason, in this chapter, we will briefly look at some other common addictions that affect drug addicts.

Co-dependency

While co-dependency in and of itself is not necessarily classed as an addiction, co-dependent traits can be addictive and are extremely dysfunctional. There many grey areas when attempting to diagnose co-dependence, because it is very hard to detect unless you are in recovery from co-dependency or are aware of its typical traits. For example, two people can be doing exactly the same thing at the same time, yet one of them is being co-dependent and the other is not. The simplest way to detect co-dependency is by observing the motives behind one's actions. The compulsive need to control people, circumstances and outcomes, in order to avoid feeling one's pain, is what drives co-dependent behaviour.

A co-dependent person seeks affection and approval from external sources and neglects her own well-being. Co-dependents feel flawed and unlovable. Despite the fact that in the twenty-first century we have so many more appropriate recovery support systems in place, many people in recovery often neglect their own human needs and desires. Many co-dependents are drug addicts, but many are not. A co-dependent who has never used drugs but was exposed to drug addiction in his or her family of origin is often attracted to addicts or people he or she can pity who need 'fixing'.

The greatest gift you can give to someone is to be present and be a witness to their pain without trying to 'fix' them. For example, a kind woman once attended a mindfulness retreat I conducted in north Norfolk and broke down in tears after she acknowledged that she was grieving. I did not run to give her a tissue or attempt to soothe her pain. I remained in my seat and let her feel her pain. In that moment, she was able to heal a little bit more. Had I interrupted her by attempting to soothe her emotions or 'fix' her, she would have been forced to suppress her pain and would thus have ceased to grow. Whenever an adult breaks down and weeps or verbally expresses that he or she is in emotional pain, it is much healthier to let that person feel his or her suffering. In other words, let an adult feel so that he or she can heal.

Love addiction

Love addicts essentially use romantic relationships to 'fix' their frozen emotional pain and mental suffering. Love addiction, like other addictive behaviours, often stems from a lack of sufficient emotional nourishment in infancy and adolescence. It leaves love addicts feeling incomplete, abandoned, flawed and unable to give or receive love in a healthy way.

Love addicts often confuse sex with love. They believe that sex is an expression of being loved. In a different context, making love can be an expression of true love (not addicted co-dependent 'love'), but a love addict who has not grieved her original pain will go through life mistaking sex for love.

Love addicts are often hooked on falling in love. They easily mistake 'falling in love' with 'mature love'. A romantic partner to a love addict is like a syringe to a heroin addict and 'falling in love' is the ultimate high. The love addict has realized that she can get high on the euphoric, exciting and sexual emotions that rush through her body as a result of falling in love. During this period, there is explosive sexual chemistry and a sense of deep unity between the two people in the relationship. This warm, fuzzy emotional state usually only lasts 12–18 months, however, and is a result of brain chemistry. After 18 months the high level of sexual tension and testosterone returns to a steady and normal rate. Sooner or later the couple start to see each other's shortcomings and reality kicks in.

Many people in a relationship at this stage often say, 'I love my husband, but I'm not "in love" with him any more' or 'I love my girlfriend, but I don't feel as intensely about her as when we first met.' Many relationships tend to end at this point or a distance develops between the couple. At this stage, the couple have an opportunity to mature into a deeper, loving relationship. Making love, for couples who have gone through the 'in love' stage, tends to become much more enjoyable if the relationship continues and if both parties are emotionally well. Unfortunately, many love addicts and love avoidants miss this opportunity to develop a deeper, more meaningful relationship and simply move on in search of the next high.

Love addicts often indulge in sexual or romantic intrigue to deliberately alter their mood. The female love addict may fantasize about being rescued by a 'hero' and compulsively look for such a man, using her sexual powers to seduce him. She will quickly realize, however, that the man she seduced cannot fulfil her need to be loved and validated. A love addict who starts to feel the effects of falling in love fading away will either end the relationship and move on to someone else to recapture the 'love high' or will stay in the relationship and desperately try to resuscitate the euphoria. A male love addict may fantasize about a woman who can unconditionally nurture him and give him bountiful sexual intercourse.

The love addict who stays with her partner after the love high has dissipated will often become obsessive. She cannot afford to lose her emotional security blanket to external forces, otherwise the buried feelings of abandonment and trauma from childhood will surface again – to face those feelings is unbearable for a love addict who does not have a non-shaming support network. While the dream of being in a relationship with 'a hero' starts to fade away, the love addict might become extremely jealous and defensive or might act out in extreme ways to give the relationship some sort of a jolt, to gain the full attention of the love avoidant. This may take the form of a violent argument to orchestrate 'make-up' sex or may entail another way of creating a drama, to the extremes of threatening to self-harm or even commit suicide if the addict's partner leaves. The primary goal of the love addict is to deny or escape from his or her suppressed feelings of grave abandonment.

Love addicts sometimes stay in a dysfunctional relationship for years because the chaos of the relationship is similar to that of their upbringing and is therefore familiar. By and large, a love addict tends to be attracted to a love avoidant. While the love addict tends to give 'all of herself' to her partner, the love avoidant pushes intimacy away and creates barriers to stop the love addict from 'controlling him'. Both men and women can be love addicts and similarly, both men and women can be love avoidants. The irony of a love addict chasing a love avoidant is that the love addict is actually recreating the hurt and abandonment that started in childhood. When the love addict grieves his or her pain and childhood losses, the momentum of love addiction fades away and self-care and self-compassion can become the foundation for building a new life in recovery. Similarly, when the love avoidant faces the deep losses tucked away in his or her body and consciousness, he or she can start to trust again and practise self-care.

Emotional, sexual and social anorexia

Many people who come into recovery for love addiction and love avoidance discover that they are emotionally anorexic, meaning that they starve themselves of emotional nourishment. In the Sex and Love Addicts Anonymous twelve-step programme (Sex and Love Addicts Anonymous, n.d.), anorexia is described in the following terms: 'As an eating disorder, anorexia is defined as the compulsive avoidance of food. In the area of sex and love, anorexia has a similar definition: Anorexia is the compulsive avoidance of giving or receiving social, sexual or emotional nourishment.'

Like emotional and sexual anorexia, social anorexia is very common among people with addictive behaviours. It is very easy for addicts to isolate themselves and hide behind solitary activities. A person addicted to a substance or a destructive behaviour becomes so dependent on the addiction to temporarily mask his emotional pain that when he gets into recovery, he often feels terribly exposed at the thought of a social gathering.

By and large, workaholics are probably those most affected by social anorexia. They lock themselves away in the workplace or take refuge in their career of choice.

Pornography and cyber-sex addiction

Dr Valerie Voon, of the University of Cambridge, has scanned the brains of pornography addicts using fMRI and found significant differences when she compared them to those of people who have not viewed online pornography (University of Cambridge, 2014). The changes were very similar to the alterations that occur in the brains of chemically dependent people. Gary Wilson gives a frank account of the high-speed online porn epidemic in his book *Your Brain on Porn* (2015). The use of pornography can also cause problems with sexual health and relationships. Many addicts, both male and female, report being indifferent to whether they have sex with their partners or not as they find that 'real' sex has become mundane.

Gambling addiction

Due to the greater availability of instant-access gambling sites, gambling addiction is on the rise. In the twentieth century, a compulsive gambler would have to make his or her way to a local bookmaker to bet on the horses or visit an arcade with multiple slot machines. Some had financial accounts with big gambling companies and could make advance bets on the telephone. In the digital age, however, an addict can gamble on his phone within seconds and find a constant stream of online gambling apps offering a 'free bet'. Gambling addiction, which is a process addiction, may also alter brain activity. A win while gambling releases a dopamine hit and a loss causes a compulsion to repeat the process.

Gambling addiction causes immense suffering and can lead to poverty, bankruptcy, divorce and family break- down. As a result of working in addiction treatment rehabs, I have witnessed first-hand the devastating effects gambling addiction can have on families.

Many drug addicts have problems with gambling. Even if a drug addict practises total abstinence with regard to using mind- and mood-altering drugs, she may maintain or develop a gambling addiction. In the world of major peak performance sportspeople, gambling addiction is catching up with alcohol addiction and, in some cases, overtaking it.

Compulsive underearning

According to Underearners Anonymous (2017):

> Underearning is many things, not all of which are about money. While the most visible consequence is the inability to provide for one's needs, including future needs, underearning is also about the inability to fully acknowledge and express our capabilities and competencies. It is about underachieving, or under-being, no matter how much money we make.

Essentially, underearning means 'hiding' and there is an element of underbeing – neglecting one's mental, emotional, physical, spiritual and financial well-being (to survive rather than thrive). It has been said that compulsive underearners are like gravely wounded animals. Rather than being out on the field with other animals to supply for its own needs, the underearner hides away in a cave, terrified of being hurt and abused. Isolation and feeling 'frozen' in the ability to earn money regularly and sufficiently, and to be positively visible, are common traits of underearners. Chronic fear, toxic shame, toxic guilt and anxiety also drive compulsive underearning.

Compulsive underearners often undervalue their services and goods. Most underearners have a very hard time creating steady or multiple sources of income.

A compulsive underearner retreats when it comes to building more prosperity, even if he dearly wishes to expand his work and live more prosperously. Stability boredom, defensiveness and self-sabotage are common traits of a compulsive underearner.

Compulsive underearning is not just about a lack of material wealth. The lack of a regular sufficient income is a result of chronic dysfunctional behaviour and a warped perception with regard to being fully self-supporting and living an abundant and prosperous life. Many compulsive underearners become compulsive debtors too.

By and large, compulsive underearners are terrified of being visible. They fear being criticized or having their work taken away from them if they become too successful (this is often a symptom of unhealed trauma from child-hood). Compulsive underearners (even those who are wealthy) are often carrying trauma and chronic shame and low self-worth. The opposite of compulsive under-earning and underbeing is to be positively visible, to live gracefully and abundantly, which is possible in recovery.

5

Mindfulness and the brain

What is mindfulness?

Essentially, 'mindfulness' means having a deeper awareness of what *is*. Mindfulness entails being aware of our thoughts, feelings and body sensations as they arise in the present moment. When we practise mindfulness in everyday life, we can observe our brain activity, witness our thought patterns and survival traits. We can be aware of our strengths and personal assets. Mindfulness can help us to access pure awareness and enhance our spiritual development.

There are many different ways to be mindful in everyday life. We can be mindful of the feelings in our bodies while we eat or walk. We can train ourselves to listen deeply to another person's words and feelings. Practices such as deep breathing, conscious breathing, alternate breathing, singing and dancing, laughing and chanting mantras can anchor us in the present moment. Sometimes we may feel serene and joyful after sitting quietly and meditating, but most of the time mindfulness produces greater clarity in one's thought patterns and emotions.

A recent Harvard study has shown that people dedicated to mindfulness have rebuilt the grey matter in their brains. Sara Lazar, of the MGH Psychiatric Neuro-imaging Research Program, a Harvard Medical School instructor in psychology, says (McGreevey, 2011):

> Although the practice of meditation is associated with a sense of peacefulness and physical relaxation, practitioners have long claimed that meditation also provides cognitive and psychological benefits that persist throughout the day. This study demonstrates that changes in brain structure may underlie some of these reported improvements and that people are not just feeling better because they are spending time relaxing.

Identifying feelings

People who carry unhealed emotional pain often develop compulsive and irrational reactive behaviours or coping mechanisms. They may have many talents but their wounded self sabotages any chance of making progress in their lives. For example, a woman with a compulsive personality might be a very quick thinker but, conversely, she will regularly lose her temper over trivial matters.

What we call emotional intelligence is a reflection of having self-awareness and being mindful of one's thoughts, feelings, beliefs, triggers and addictive reactive patterns. Being able to detect how one is truly feeling in the present moment and articulating that to others is a sign of emotional intelligence. Generally speaking, emotional intelligence in adulthood develops during the process of grief work or deep feeling work. Those who dedicate themselves to learning and applying the emotional literacy that comes with emotional intelligence have usually gone through a series of crushing blows in their personal or emotional lives. Of course, many are fortunate enough to have been brought up in a home that encouraged talking regularly about one's feelings and moods. Only then can we have greater clarity with regard to communicating with others. The more we can label and process our feelings, the easier it is to be authentic.

We may be aware of all sorts of moods and emotions that appear and dissolve in the human body. See if you can identify any of the following emotions as ones that you experience in your everyday life:

- anger
- anxiety
- joy
- happiness
- cheerfulness
- apathy
- rage
- resentment
- arousal
- worry
- anticipation
- contentment
- hope
- guilt
- loneliness
- lust
- envy
- jealousy
- boredom
- excitement
- contempt
- desire
- curiosity
- fear
- gratitude
- appreciation
- sadness
- sorrow
- despair
- embarrassment
- humiliation
- wonder
- bliss

On reflection, are you able to see that there is much more to you than a particular mood? Can you see how quickly your mood can change?

The more we can immediately identify what we are feeling, the more we can temper our behaviour.

Mindful breathing exercises

Nasal breathing enhances clarity, memory and learning. Meditators have manipulated the breath to access inner peace and contentment for over three thousand years, and modern-day science is also revealing the health benefits for the brain of nasal breathing. Consciously breathing through your nostrils (and being aware of the inhale breath) can improve your emotional health, as well as your capacity to learn and make better emotional judgements.

Through several fascinating experiments at North-western University in Illinois, scientists have proved that nasal breathing can activate electrical brain signals that lead to improved memory and cognitive processes. Christina Zelano, Assistant Professor of Neurology at the university's Feinberg School of Medicine, has commented (Paul, 2016):

> One of the major findings in this study is that there is a dramatic difference in brain activity in the amygdala and hippocampus during inhalation compared with exhalation. When you breathe in, we discovered you are stimulating neurons in the olfactory cortex, amygdala and hippocampus, all across the limbic system.

Conscious nasal breathing, therefore, can calm us down and reduce anxiety and stress. The scientists at Northwestern University found that breathing through the nostrils had a bigger positive impact on the human brain than breathing through the mouth. Furthermore, inhaling through the nostrils had a more powerful effect on the brain than exhaling through the nostrils.

The experiments were inspired by scientists' findings when they monitored patients with epilepsy and studied their brains as a result of a surgeon implanting electrodes to discover what originally caused the seizures. The results showed that brain activity changed as a result of breathing, particularly in the amygdala and hippocampus – regions of the brain where feelings and sensations are processed. This prompted more discussion and curiosity about the power of the breath and, consequently, the Northwestern scientists carried out a study of 60 people. The subjects were asked to look at photos of people with surprised or fearful facial expressions and identify instantaneously which emotion each face was expressing.

The subjects noticed that, while inhaling, they could identify a fearful facial expression more rapidly than when they exhaled. This was not the case when the subjects viewed surprised facial expressions, however. This indicates that nature has provided *Homo sapiens* with the means to increase our chances of survival by being able to quickly identify potential threats and that consciously inhaling can give us greater clarity in dangerous situations. This can also help us to read other people's painful facial expressions while developing our own emotional intelligence.

In another experiment focused on the hippocampus, the same 60 people were shown a variety of objects on a computer screen and asked to remember and say what they saw afterwards. The scientists found that the subjects were able to remember what the objects were with greater clarity if they viewed the objects while inhaling than when they were exhaling. This means that we can deliberately choose to inhale while absorbing important information.

Mindfulness as the cornerstone for healing trauma

In my personal recovery, mindfulness has helped me to become aware of my trauma responses and given me an anchor to stay present when I have been triggered. Being able to feel my triggers without reacting must be largely credited to learning to anchor myself in my body through mindful body scan meditation. Triggers can happen randomly and they would often cause an emotional eruption until I came to terms with my trauma and practised mindfulness daily. Similarly, I have met scores of people recovering from addictive behaviour who have been able to make peace with their trauma and their triggers as a result of making mindfulness a way of life.

A mindfulness-based approach to anxiety disorders and phobias

While prescribed medicine is still a solution for many people with anxiety disorders and phobias, medical doctors in the West have recognized the remarkable benefits of practising mindfulness in order to relieve symptoms of these conditions. People in recovery from the use of mind- and mood-altering substances may want to be very careful what substances they put into their system; I myself made a conscious choice to use mindfulness and yoga to address my anxiety. Some people do need medication, however, and they should certainly consult their doctor.

Personally, I find breathing techniques such as alternate breathing (pranayama yoga), deep breathing, mindful walking and observing the breath are very effective in settling my anxiety. I used to suffer regular panic attacks that were heightened as a result of substance misuse. The paradox is that when I feel my anxious emotions without numbing out and attempting to suppress them, the anxiety dissolves and therefore I am liberated from it. Many people have reported a similar experience: when they feel their anxiety without distraction, they eventually become less anxious. Thankfully, there are many different methods of addressing anxiety disorders and phobias today and help can be sought without fear of being 'judged'.

One day at a time, one moment at a time

Many emotionally wounded people subconsciously make 'control' their primary religion. They become obsessed with manipulating outcomes and create absurd expectations of themselves and others. Pathologically obsessing about controlling the future can lead to chronic stress, one of the biggest killers in our species. Too much stress can cause inflammation, short-term memory loss and heart disease, to name but a few.

Thankfully, when we anchor ourselves in the moment we can greatly reduce this stress. Living one day at a time releases everyday pressures. Living one day at a time does not mean that we neglect planning or preparing for future events. It simply means that we anchor ourselves in the present day – thus the saying 'just for today'. To go a step further, it is even more fruitful to anchor ourselves in the present moment. When we approach the day with an awareness of 'one day at a time, one moment at a time', everyday life becomes more manageable. The reality, of course, is that we only ever have this moment. Therefore, if we are grounded in the present, we are centred in reality.

Box breathing and monitoring the breath

Learn how to breathe properly and monitor the flow of your breathing as often as possible. During a stressful moment, see if you can catch yourself taking short breaths (shallow breathing). This is a good time to pause and take several deep breaths, inhaling through the nostrils and exhaling through the mouth. A simple and practical technique I often teach professionals during my mindfulness classes and workshops is 'box breathing'. To practise box breathing, breathe in for four seconds through the nostrils. Hold your breath for four seconds. Then breathe out through your mouth for four seconds. Hold your breath once more for four seconds. Repeat this cycle for two to three minutes.

Observation of thought and primitive modes of survival

Being able to be aware that we have thoughts, but that we are not our thoughts, is a major breakthrough for people seeking emotional health and spiritual well-being. A human being will have tens of thousands of thoughts per day and, unfortunately, many of these thoughts are incredibly unkind. The danger comes when people are utterly unaware that they are not their thoughts. If an emotionally wounded person is constantly being pulled from one painful thought to another, she will feel weighed down and lose her zest for life.

It is essential to step back and monitor your thought life. What is your regular thinking pattern? What are the subtle voices and images in the mind telling you? Are you mentally directing harm inwards? Common thoughts among people recovering from suppressed grief include:

- 'He/she is mine';
- 'I hate him/her';
- 'I hate myself';
- 'I can't do it';
- 'I don't think I'll ever be able to support myself';
- 'I don't trust anyone';
- 'What's wrong with me?'

Many of our unkind thoughts towards ourselves and others operate on autopilot and, thus, they bind to constant inner and external conflict. It is important to remember that thoughts – whether kind or cruel – come and go. In recovery, we can gradually develop the habit of not being attached to every thought that randomly appears on the screen of our minds. We can learn to identify mental vitriol and say to ourselves, 'This is just another cruel thought passing through.'

Mindful brainwork

Self-directed neuroplasticity

Through self-directed neuroplasticity we can make a conscious choice to rewire our brains, one day at a time, one moment at a time. With every experience, thought, feeling, sensation and environment we are exposed to, we are literally changing and rewiring the human brain. One of the world's leading experts on neuroplasticity, Dr Jeffrey M. Schwartz, has taught that the human brain is a phenomenal plastic organ that we can shape by using our human will and regularly absorbing a functional, non-shaming environment. As co-author with me of *The Kindness Habit* (2016, p. 46), Dr Barbara Mariposa has written, 'The brain is changing and responding moment by moment. New inputs create new neural connections and pathways – new learning – all the time.' For people recovering from drug addiction and emotional wounds, this means that we can consciously change our lives. For example, the idea of self-directed neuroplasticity means we can use our human will and a deep desire to behave in a new way, regardless of how uncomfortable or emotionally painful it may feel.

New experiences change your neural network

In their book *Super Brain* (2013), Deepak Chopra and Rudolph Tanzi show how self-awareness, mindfulness, plenty of sleep and a healthy diet can improve our brain health and reduce memory loss, anxiety, stress and depression. Spiritual and emotional recovery are possible because the human brain is a living organ that we can transform by making new choices and being in non-shaming recovery-based environments. When we have new experiences that inspire us, we are literally painting a new and wonderful reality. We can create new neural pathways that enhance our emotional well-being by changing our environment and by learning to be present.

A personal inventory for utilizing your brain

1 Do you consciously put time aside every day to rewire your brain?

2 Do you consciously expose yourself to new creative and intellectual experiences to change your neural network?

3 How often do you change your environment and meet new people who inspire you and challenge you to raise your capacity to serve the greater good?

4 Are you prepared to consciously integrate your brain-stem, limbic area and pre-frontal cortex by practising mindfulness daily?

5 If you have come to terms with the fact that you are shut off from your creative spontaneous spark, are you prepared to consciously work on strengthening the creative parts of your brain?

6 How aware are you with regard to your regular thought patterns, mental monologues, feelings and perhaps addictive behaviours?

7 On average, how often do you practise mindfulness meditation and/or other mindful practices?

8 Are you able to emotionally anchor yourself in the day and still plan for the future? In other words, can you practise 'one day at a time'?

6

Your sacred inner child

We did not come into this world loathing ourselves or wishing to numb our feelings. As small children, we operated from a place of wonder, curiosity, spontaneity and creativity. As an infant, it was easy to find a sense of awe at the sight of a star in the sky or appreciate a bumblebee buzzing away in the great outdoors. We could see the humanness in all people without being drenched in tribal, fearful and prejudiced concepts. There was an unconditional acceptance of the nowness of life.

Unfortunately, many children's spirits are eclipsed by constant careless remarks, verbal, physical or sexual abuse and chronic toxic shame in a family home. How many children lose hope and their sense of wonder because they have grown up in an environment that is riddled with untreated mental illness, drug addiction and other grave addictive behaviours? How many adults are alive today who have lost any sense of their true self, as a result of carrying frozen wounds from childhood? When a child's spirit is crushed, the same child will develop dysfunctional survival traits that can be highly problematic in adulthood. The child, now a fully grown adult, is emotionally immature, regardless of demonstrating self-reliance.

I believe that there is a sacred child-like spirit in all of us (often referred to as our younger self or sacred inner child), one we can access and heal in recovery. We can gradually learn to integrate our youthful spirit into our everyday life. There is sweet sacredness when a person truly dedicates himself or herself to reclaiming his or her forgotten and abandoned inner child. When the inner child is integrated with the adult self, life becomes fulfilling, abundant and fruitful.

The concept of the inner child

Adult Children of Alcoholics and Dysfunctional Families (formerly Adult Children of Alcoholics), a twelve-step fellowship founded in 1977–78, has integrated the concept of the inner child throughout the very fabric of its twelve-step programme. On several occasions in the fellowship's red book, the authors use the terms 'inner child' and 'true self' to describe the same idea.

The concept of the inner child – and, more precisely, 'the wounded inner child' – was popularized internationally in the 1980s by John Bradshaw. In 1990, Bradshaw published an instant number one *New York Times* bestseller,

Homecoming (Little, Brown, 1991), which, as its subtitle clearly states, is concerned with 'reclaiming and championing your inner child'.

In 1991, Lucia Capacchione's important book on the inner child was published, *Recovery of Your Inner Child* (Simon & Schuster, 1991). Capacchione's professional approach focuses on writing and drawing with the non-dominant hand and on creative journaling. Her work stands her in good stead as a pioneer of healing the inner child through the expressive arts.

John Bradshaw's *Homecoming*

Homecoming by John Bradshaw is one of the most profound recovery books I have ever studied. It helps the reader to reclaim his or her inner child and heal frozen emotional wounds through gentle step-by-step exercises.

Bradshaw believes that by revisiting childhood and consciously seeking to nurture and heal the wounded inner child, the adult will gain a new meaning from life and a deeper fulfilment. He identifies five primary stages in reclaiming the inner child:

- infant inner child
- toddler inner child
- preschooler inner child
- school inner child
- adolescent inner child.

According to Bradshaw, when we carefully integrate all these five compartments of our wounded inner child and give them the unconditional love that they have been denied, we can become whole and therefore authentic.

Accessing your inner child – ways to connect

Collecting photos of your inner child

It can be very therapeutic to keep several photos of your younger self; put them next to your morning meditation books or in a place where you typically sit in silence once a day. By looking regularly at photos of yourself as a child and assuring him or her that he or she is not forgotten and is loved, you can ground yourself in the present moment and heal. Sometimes you might feel inspired to write a letter to your inner child after looking at a photo of yourself (we will cover this in the next section). If you have a photo of yourself as an infant, look into the eyes of the child and notice the innocence. That innocence is still inside you; it is your humanness. If you are unable to access a photo of yourself when you were younger, then visualize yourself as a small child and be fully aware of the innocence this child carried with him or her. Then sense that this purity was once easy for you to access without the fear of being rejected and hurt.

A letter to your inner child

An effective way to connect with your sacred inner child is to write him or her a handwritten letter (avoid using a mobile phone, laptop or computer). After you have written a letter to your inner child, wait and see if something inside you feels to be responding to the letter you have written. Do not try and force the process, but nonetheless keep the pen and paper near you. If you sense that a written response will come through you, reply using your non-dominant hand.

If this is the first time that your inner child has written back to you, distressing revelations may manifest. It is important that you do not try to guess what your younger self is trying to communicate with you. You do not need to fill in the blanks and write what you think your inner child ought to be saying. Gentleness and patience is essential when communicating with your vulnerable and hurt younger self. Make sure to give yourself some privacy when writing. If possible, make an effort to write to your younger self at least once a week. This act of self-care will empower you.

Sacred inner child guided meditation

To help you maximize your deep feeling work, I have written an inner child guided meditation for you to use. All you need is an audio recorder. If you have a mobile phone with a voice recorder app, that will be sufficient. Simply read the guided meditation script out loud, recording your own voice. When you have finished reading out the script, stop recording and then make sure you have some privacy to listen back to the recording. Sit with the emotions you feel after listening to the meditation. Last, if possible, sit in a comfortable position before you begin to meditate.

Sacred inner child guided meditation

Close your eyes.

Notice that you are breathing without any effort on your part. Be aware of the air that flows within and through you. Feel the breath move in and out of your body. Notice how you inhale and how you exhale effortlessly.

Pause recording for 30 seconds.

Observe the body breathing. Feel the breath enter your body. Feel the breath leave your body. Notice how your chest and tummy rise as you breathe effortlessly. Continue watching the breath.

Pause recording for 30 seconds.

Now remember a time in your childhood. A time when you were very young. A time when you were still enthusiastic about seeing new things like a flower or a bird flying through the air. See yourself during this time of innocence, playfulness and sweetness.

Pause recording for 20 seconds.

Now see this innocent child playing in a park on a bright, warm and sunny day. See the child laughing at the birds hopping about as they come closer to the swing.

Pause recording for 20 seconds.

Now see your parents or carers walking towards the child in the park. Notice how the child feels the closer the parents come towards the swing. Notice the child's facial expressions.

Pause recording for 20 seconds.

Now see yourself, as a fully grown adult, calmly walking towards the child and your parents. See yourself walking with confidence and at a casual pace.

Pause recording for 20 seconds.

As you approach the child and your parents, see the child notice you. See how the child looks at you and how your parents turn round to look at you. Notice how you walk right up to the swing. Hear yourself say to the child, 'What a lovely smile.' Notice how your parents' body language takes a defensive stance, while the child looks at you in awe.

Pause recording for 20 seconds.

Look your parents in the eye and calmly say to them, 'Thank you for looking after my inner child but it's time that he/she came home with me. I am taking my inner child back and he/she will not be coming here again.' Now pick up your inner child and give him/her a kiss on the cheek. Say goodbye to your parents and turn around with the child in your arms. Notice how your inner child is gripping on to you. Your inner child feels safe around you. Now calmly walk away from the park and your parents. Remember that you are in control, not your parents.

Pause recording for 20 seconds.

As you continue walking in the opposite direction, comfort your inner child and tell him/her that you love him/her so much and, from now on, you are going to parent him/her. Assure your inner child that you are going to love and accept him/her unconditionally.

Pause recording for 20 seconds.

Now see yourself and your inner child walk up some steps away from the park. Start to climb the hill with the child. Notice how clear the blue sky is and how brightly the sun is shining. Be aware of how your inner child is in awe of nature and laughs when a bird flies close to the two of you. Continue walking with the child.

Pause recording for 20 seconds.

Finally, look your inner child in the eye and see his/her authenticity radiate from his/her face. See yourself in the child. Now let the child see him/herself in you.

Pause recording for 20 seconds.

Now take five deep breaths. On the inhale breath, count to seven. On the exhale breath, count to seven. After taking five deep breaths, open your eyes and sit with your feelings for a few minutes.

Stop recording.

After you have completed the inner child guided meditation, write down with a pen in a journal what you were feeling during the meditation. What emotions came up? For example, did you shed any tears?

Respecting your inner child's truth

When you have rekindled your sacred inner child, a desire to explore a new reality will emerge. Almost immediately after reconnecting with my inner child (my authentic self), I had an overwhelming desire to start gardening, so I spent the spring and summer digging up the soil and planting flowers and herbs. As an adult, and prior to connecting with my inner child, I would avoid getting mud on my hands. My inner child, however, loves being in the garden and enjoys the texture of soil crumbling in the palms of his hands. My inner child enjoys seeing the bees working relentlessly and the fragrance of a lily or a red rose. Furthermore, my inner child has given me an even deeper reverence for the great outdoors and nature.

In hindsight, my inner child has been gradually re-appearing since I got clean and sober in the summer of 2004. For example, I became a vegetarian in the summer of 2013. In the summer of 2017, I became a vegan. I realize that my inner child never liked eating meat or dairy. My inner child loves plant-based meals.

Mindfully being in the moment

Fun activities to do with your inner child

There are all sorts of activities to do to supplement your inner child's desire to play. In my view, it is important to put time aside on a regular basis and find fun things to do. Healthy fun and play time is essential in recovery. The problem is that many of us do not know how to have healthy fun. Writing a letter to your inner child and asking him or her what he or she considers to be fun is one way of gaining more clarity if you get stuck and cannot think of any good ideas.

After writing the letter from your adult self, wait for a response from your inner child – but remember not to force a written response. And if you feel that your inner child is going to communicate with you through a written response, remember to write with your non-dominant hand. My inner child finds joy being around animals, in the great outdoors, go-karting and canoeing, and likes to paint. For example, when I commit to putting a couple of hours aside to paint, sometimes I can create three or four paintings. I usually paint with my non-dominant hand, which fills me with joy and stops me from trying to paint a 'perfect picture'. Similarly, some of my fellow travellers in recovery enjoy going skiing, cycling, surfing and roller-skating.

Paint a picture of your inner child

The final exercise in this chapter is to paint a picture (chalk or colouring pens/pencils are fine) of the concept of an inner child. Paint the picture with your non-dominant hand and see what happens. There should be no outcome in mind. You might end up with paint all over your fingers and blotches of different colours in your picture or else a more specific image might manifest. Unearthed feelings and memories might appear.

If possible, put time aside regularly to paint and draw. It is a good way to stay connected to your inner child. Once you get into a regular flow of painting or drawing for the sake of it, you might find that new areas of your creativity expand and unfold.

7

Mindful ways to enhance self-respect

Becoming aware of self-critical voices in our minds

Before coming into recovery, many of us were particularly cruel to ourselves by directing vitriol inwards. Our cruel thoughts fed off our static emotional pain. Below are some of the common and universal mean-spirited thoughts that fester and recycle in emotionally wounded people's minds. Remember that these destructive thought patterns are shame-based and do not reflect our true selves. See if you can recognize any of them in your own belief system.

- 'I'm an imposter.'
- 'I'm unlovable.'
- 'I'm flawed.'
- 'I hate myself.'
- 'It's just a matter of time before everything collapses and goes horribly wrong.'

MINDFUL WAYS TO ENHANCE SELF-RESPECT **97**

- 'Evil will have the last say.'
- 'There is no justice in this world.'
- 'I'll never be good enough.'
- 'What's the point?'
- 'I need to be perfect to be accepted.'
- 'If I can control my life, I'll feel better about myself.'
- 'I can't trust anyone. People will always let me down.'
- 'What's wrong with me?'
- 'I'm so stupid.'

Stop saying 'Sorry'!

Compulsively saying 'Sorry' is often a reflection of wanting to apologize for our very existence. I used to say the word 'sorry' when there was no need for me to do so. It became a habit and reflected my chronic toxic shame, low self-worth and low self-esteem. Generally speaking, shame-based people will even apologize when someone else has harmed them. For example, a woman with low self-worth walks along a busy road and a man looking at his mobile phone rather than watching where he is going bumps into her. The man glued to his mobile phone carries on walking as though nothing has happened while the woman he has barged into apologizes.

My fellows and I in recovery made a joint decision to stop overusing the word 'sorry'. Every now and then, however, I still catch myself apologizing without just cause. For instance, while walking into a church hall recently to attend a recovery support group, I noticed that the main church hall was hosting a pantomime. There was a long queue of people lined up from the entrance to the kitchen next to the room where the support group was meeting. For some reason, I had an unwelcome feeling of being an imposter (a shame attack) and instead of saying 'Excuse me', I said, 'Sorry'. A man responded, saying that there was no need to say sorry. He was right and he reminded me to honour my self-worth.

Feeling inferior or superior to others

Feeling inferior or superior to any other human being is a mirage; usually a manifestation of low self-worth. I find that feeling superior to anyone at a human level quickly leads to feeling superior to a particular group of people and that can lead to dehumanization. Equally, feeling inferior harms our self-worth.

While someone else might develop certain skills that I cannot replicate, it does not mean that I am 'less than' that person as a human being. It is extremely unlikely that I am going to be able to build a giant corporation like Microsoft or be in a position to give away billions of dollars. While I respect and celebrate Bill Gates's wonderful contribution to our species and to the planet, there is no reason for me to feel inferior to him at a human level. In other words, developing a fine skill set or calculating one's net worth is not to be confused with one's self-worth.

Some people are addicted to hero-worshipping. They put someone on a pedestal until they realize that that person too is human. As a result they quickly find someone new to idolize. While hero-worshipping may be common in adolescence, if such behaviour continues in adulthood it can become dysfunctional. When hero-worshipping another human being we cut ourselves off from our authentic selves. For people who lack it, the process of enhancing their true self-worth brings with it the unravelling of their survival behaviours. It becomes unattractive to us to put people on a pedestal or to look down at others. To do so is to deny our own humanness.

Healing from people pleasing

People pleasing and putting others first literally diminished my mental, emotional, spiritual and physical well-being. Overwhelmingly, most emotionally wounded people demonstrate this trait. Many of us have been programmed to put others first; to be of service to others before we serve ourselves. While being of service to others is essential if we are to properly integrate into society, being of service to ourselves first is more important.

Unfortunately, I developed the habit of thinking that I had to please people in order to be accepted, liked and loved. I thought that if I neglected my own well-being to please a work colleague, employer or fair-weather friend, I would get on well in this world. Sadly, however, it did not work out that way. I took on way too many professional projects and overlooked the necessity to sleep properly. At one point, I was giving money to charity when I needed the extra cash myself because I didn't know how to manage the feelings of pity and guilt I experienced when I was approached by charities.

All this dysfunctional behaviour was a result of believing that other people's needs were more important than my own. I have had many conversations with fellow ex-people pleasers who have had similar experiences. They didn't have the courage to say 'No' to a highly dysfunctional family member who was begging for money to buy drugs or to gamble. They didn't have the courage to say 'No' when they didn't feel like having sex. They didn't have the courage to say 'No' when people asked them for 'favours'. They often associated with people they pitied. To compound the problem, they couldn't even say 'Yes' when a friend offered them a holiday home abroad for free because they didn't want to impose themselves. Some men and women have shared that they stayed in a marriage because they didn't want to break their partner's heart.

There is another price to pay for being a people pleaser. It means that we cannot truly be ourselves. If we say 'No' when we mean 'Yes' and 'Yes' when we mean 'No', we are creating a false sense of self. We develop the habit of being dishonest with ourselves and others. This can only lead to deep resentment and unhappiness. It is a tragedy to go through life not knowing who we are and neglecting our true self in this way.

If you are a people pleaser and tend to put others' needs above your own to such an extent that you are seething with resentment, you can stop this destructive and counterproductive behaviour. The next time you find yourself in the midst of people pleasing, take a deep breath and pause for a moment. Recognize the tendency to neglect your well-being and begin to take care of yourself, there and then. At first it might feel 'wrong' to put your own needs first and to honour your personal well-being, but it gets easier with practice.

Uncovering and developing your core values

It is not possible to demonstrate our own values if we are chronic people pleasers. To live by our values means that we are going to come up against resistance once in a while – and perhaps more often. The idea of one's values being challenged and mocked can be a terrifying prospect for an emotionally wounded person, particularly for an addict afraid of people. The person hiding feels that it is a safer option to try and please everyone, but the price he pays for this miscalculation is very high indeed. The price is a loss of integrity, dignity and self-empowerment.

When we grow out of people pleasing we gain much more clarity with regard to our true values; we get in touch with our core authentic beliefs about who we are and how we view the world. We can stand up for our core beliefs and speak up if necessary, feeling good for doing so.

A helpful way to get in touch with your values is to write them down on a piece of paper (or on your computer). Why not write out your core human values and see if you are honouring them in your everyday life? What do you feel strongly about? What do you really believe in? Keep in mind that developing and honouring values is a process and no one can demonstrate perfection in this area.

Writing an affirming letter to your wounded self

Writing a letter to affirm your place on Earth can complement your emotional recovery. Therefore the next exercise is to write a letter to your wounded self and let him or her know that he or she is safe, loved and cared for and no longer needs to believe he or she is not good enough. After you have written a letter to your wounded self, see if something inside of you feels able to respond. If you feel that a written response will come through you, reply using your non-dominant hand. Below is a short example.

Dear X,

It's important that you know I am here for you. I know how much you have suffered and how much pain you have had to keep to yourself. I understand the shame you have stored and carried for so many years.

I want you to know that you have a right to be alive. I accept your wounds and pain. I accept that you are imperfect and I celebrate your humanness. Whenever your pain starts to overwhelm you, I will be here to reassure you that you are not alone. I love you.

Warmly,
X

A guided self-worth meditation

I have written this guided self-worth meditation for you to record and play back to yourself. Simply read out loud the text below and record your own voice until the end of the script. When you have finished reading the meditation out loud, stop recording and then make sure you have some quiet time to listen back to it. Sit with the emotions you feel after listening to the recording.

A guided self-worth meditation

Close your eyes.

Notice that you are breathing without any effort on your part. Be aware of the air that flows within and through you. Feel the breath move in and out of your body. Notice how you inhale and how you exhale effortlessly.

Pause recording for 30 seconds.

Observe your body breathing. Feel the breath enter your body. Feel the breath leave your body. Notice how your chest and tummy rise as you breathe effortlessly. Continue watching the breath.

Pause recording for 30 seconds.

I know your deepest secret. I feel this secret at the core of my being. I have felt it for many years. I know that you feel that you are unlovable and unworthy of life. I know that you have blamed yourself for the abuse inflicted on you. You have felt responsible for your family of origin's problems and hurts. You blamed yourself when they acted inappropriately towards you. You took it all on and as a result, you feel like a failure. I know what it feels like to be toxically shamed and abused.

I know what it feels like to be fighting your corner every day and feeling you have to affirm to our species that you are deserving of a place on Earth. I know what it feels like to have many buttons that people press on a regular basis and I know how terribly lonely it is to feel defective and ugly inside.

I just want you to know that these emotions are not your fault. You were not born with these emotions. Your carers and warped aspects of society handed on false perceptions to you when you were innocent and unable to defend yourself. You are in fact worthy of being alive. You are worthy of being a part of the human species. No one is more important than you. No one is less important than you. Your life, like every single human life, is of equal value.

Pause recording for 20 seconds.

From now on whenever I feel your pain and shame, I will be here to remind you that I love you and you are OK just the way you are. I will remind you that it is natural to make mistakes and that just because you make an error it does not mean that you are a mistake. When I feel that you have been triggered by someone, I will promptly reassure you that you are in safe hands.

Pause recording for 20 seconds.

To protect you, from now on I will only seek fellowship with people who are safe and have emotional boundaries. If you are troubled by someone I meet or work with in a professional setting, rest assured I will exercise strong boundaries around this person.

    I will practise self-care and put our needs first. I will make a conscious effort not to people please, seeing that there is no reason to people please any more. I will consciously let go of being a victim or a victimizer. I am here for you until we draw our last breath.

Love,
X

Now take several deep breaths.

Stop recording.

8

Healing the pain of betrayal and abandonment

Trust issues

Emotionally wounded addicts have an extremely difficult time with intimacy and with trusting themselves and others. They have a deep desire to trust, but their emotional scars and traumatic memories haunt them whenever an opportunity to trust another person arises. Naturally this can lead to a very lonely existence. The challenge is to take the first step by reaching out to a professional or a warm-hearted support group and revealing oneself. Unless an emotionally injured person begins to trust, recovery is impossible. Baby steps are often the best way when working out who is worth approaching and opening up to. The good news is that, with practice and patience, we can improve with respect to deciding who to trust and, more importantly, we can learn to trust our intuitive thoughts, feelings and hunches, as well as our own personal values.

The scars of betrayal

Betrayal can leave behind emotional scars and can prevent a person trusting altogether. Betrayal can engender cynicism and a very dark outlook on life. We all require warm fellowship, friendship and companionship. We cannot live fulfilling lives without social cohesion and a sense of belonging. The reality is that there are plenty of trustworthy people in the world rebuilding their lives. It was a very gradual process for me to open up and talk about what was really going on in my recovery. The more I started to take risks by talking to others, however, the more I had an opportunity to exercise boundaries. As I asserted new boundaries, I started to gravitate towards people with integrity, warm-heartedness and decency.

Mindful art

Paint a picture of your betrayal

Painting a picture of your betrayal will help you get in touch with your feelings of loss, sadness, isolation and abandonment. Paint your picture with your non-dominant hand and see what feelings and memories arise. There is no need to try and project an outcome before you begin. Once you have finished painting your picture, look at it for a few minutes and then jot down with a pen and paper in your journal how you feel.

Guided meditation for healing betrayal

I have put together a guided meditation for the healing of betrayal for you to record and play back to yourself. Simply read out loud the text below and record your own voice until the end of the script. When you have finished reading out the meditation, stop recording and then make sure you have some quiet time to listen back to it. Sit with the emotions you feel after listening to the recording.

Guided meditation for healing betrayal

Close your eyes.

Notice that you are breathing without any effort on your part. Be aware of the air that flows within and through you. Feel the breath move in and out of your body. Notice how you inhale and how you exhale effortlessly.

Pause recording for 30 seconds.

Observe your body breathing. Feel the breath enter and leave your body. Notice how your chest and tummy rise as you breathe effortlessly. Continue watching the life breath sustain you.

Pause recording for 20 seconds.

Now go back to a time when you felt betrayed. See the scene clearly and vividly. What is happening? Can you see the person who betrayed you? How does this make you feel? Sit with this feeling. Let yourself feel this emotion without suppressing it.

Pause recording for 20 seconds.

Now see your current True Self enter the scene and notice how the person who once betrayed you has frozen. See yourself standing up straight, expressing a relaxed and empowered body language. Notice how your betrayed self notices you and is taken aback. Now walk over to your betrayed self and say hello. Let him/her know that you are from a later life and you are here to let him/her know that he/she is not alone.

Pause recording for 20 seconds.

Ask your betrayed self to stand next to you and hold his/her hand while you both walk towards the frozen person who betrayed you. Now both you and your betrayed self look into the eyes of this person who seriously hurt you while you repeat the following words: 'You hurt and betrayed me. I have been very angry with you and I have not been able to feel entirely free because of your actions. I have carried this pain long enough, however. I have allowed you to dominate a part of my being by holding on to this hurt and I no longer wish to have this static grief in my system. I am no longer willing to abandon myself. I want you to know that what you did to me was unacceptable. Nevertheless, I am ready to let this pain be. I am willing to accept this pain that I have masked and suppressed and, by doing so, I will heal. While I might still carry the memory of your actions and while this pain might still appear in the future, just for today I am free. You cannot hurt me again. I am free.'

Pause recording for 20 seconds.

Now both of you turn around and walk away from the person who hurt you. As you walk away, put your arm around the shoulder of your betrayed self. See the two of you merge into one person and let that person look you in the eye and merge into you.

Pause recording for 20 seconds.

Now take a deep breath and feel your emotions.

Pause recording for 20 seconds.

Now take several deep breaths. Breathe in for seven seconds and breathe out for seven seconds.

Stop recording.

9

Spiritual well-being

Connecting with our personal spiritual centre

The word 'spirituality' is often associated with religion. Some confuse spirituality with spiritualism, which are two different practices altogether. While it is certainly true that many people practising a religion can have a personal spiritual centre, spirituality is not a religious matter. Each of us can explore our own personal spirituality and understanding of our inner world; our self-awareness and how we relate to nature.

Many people in recovery find that they feel spiritually grounded when in regular contact with the great outdoors. Others feel a deep serenity after lighting a candle in a church or temple or by chanting a sacred mantra. The point is that, unlike a typical religion that lays out a non-negotiable ideology, spirituality is expansive and deeply personal. The more we sincerely pray, meditate, nurture the inner child and practise spiritual principles, the more we become aware of our own awareness by observing our reality in the present moment. In moments of deep stillness during meditation we can tune in to pure awareness. We can observe our consciousness and feel at one with our fellows, with nature and the cosmos.

Spirituality allows the individual to explore and progress to higher levels of self-awareness. As we heal our major emotional wounds, personal spirituality becomes a desirable practice. In almost all universal spiritual practices, *being* is more important than ideology. It has been said by many of the world's great sages and mystical teachers that our lives are a meditation. We can be deeply aware of our life unfolding just as we can be aware of our inner world during a mindfulness meditation practice.

Stillness and spiritual bliss

Stillness and spiritual bliss can be realized in the minute gaps between periods of thought activity. For instance, when we observe and truly listen to our mental commentary, being fully aware of our own awareness, we can feel a subtle stillness. On some occasions, stillness can even lead to warm realizations of spiritual bliss. People who have been meditating daily for many years often report regularly experiencing blissful moments of transcendence and a stillness of thought.

A classic Zen story entitled 'Nansen's Ordinary Mind' illustrates the realization of stillness and spiritual bliss.

Nansen's Ordinary Mind

A student named Joshu asked his teacher, Nansen, 'What is the Way?'

Nansen glared into Joshu's eyes and replied, 'Your ordinary mind is the Way.'

Feeling slightly confused, Joshu asked, 'Can the Way be grasped?'

Nansen continued to look his student in the eye and replied, 'The more you pursue, the harder it is to realize.'

Still not satisfied with the answer, Joshu asked, 'How can I know it is the Way?'

Nansen took a deep breath and answered, 'The Way does not depend on knowledge, nor is it non-knowledge. When you realize the Way, you are free, and so how can you explain it by yes or no?'

The answer assisted Joshu in awakening and deepening his meditation practice.

Prayer and meditation

In August 2004, at the age of 21, I hit rock bottom as a result of my drug addiction. I fell on my knees weeping and cried out for help, choosing the only room in the house where there was a bronze plate depicting two hands together with an inscription reading 'God bless'. I have not had the urge to use drugs since that morning, as a result of an inner compass that reminds me never to be complacent about my personal recovery. I am not cured of addictions (that is, of addictiveness), but I have an opportunity to stay clean and sober one day a time.

Although I am not aligned with any particular religion, I do believe in a Higher Power. It is certainly possible to be totally abstinent and demonstrate a positive moral compass without believing in a Higher Power, but I personally find great comfort in prayer and expressing my gratitude to life. I feel grounded in nature and I often recite the serenity prayer several times a day.

Pure awareness and trusting our intuition

There is a difference between following your instincts and listening to your intuition. Instincts are primitive modes of survival (fight, flight, freeze, sexual urges, hunting and so on), whereas intuition is a much higher manifestation of thought and emotions. When we can be mindful of our brain activity and be consciously present, we are much more likely to tune into our intuitive nature. The more present we are, the easier it is to access pure awareness and pure consciousness and, therefore, intuitive ideas and hunches can flow through us. Intuitive feelings and insights are believed by many scientists and spiritual mystics to be a manifestation of pure awareness.

According to many sages, spiritual mystics and yogis, 'pure awareness' describes the Source of all collective and individual awareness, all modes of observation, all expression of life, consciousness and intelligence. For example, the primary awareness of a caterpillar is the primary awareness of an ape or a human being, even though their modes of observation might be completely different from one another. The thirteenth-century Persian poet Rumi famously declared, 'You are not a drop in the ocean. You are the entire ocean in a drop.' In other words, we are fundamentally pure awareness, experiencing our own individual expression of awareness.

The great sage Ramana Maharshi said (Godman, n.d.):

> You are awareness. Awareness is another name for you. Since you are awareness there is no need to attain or cultivate it. All that you have to do is to give up being aware of other things, that is of the not-self. If one gives up being aware of them then pure awareness alone remains and that is the Self.

Deepak Chopra (2014) often refers to pure awareness as God: 'God is pure awareness, in which there are multiple modes of observation, multiple perceptions.'

Maharishi Mahesh Yogi (1972), the founder of the transcendental meditation movement, explained:

> When the mind is opening to that unbounded pure awareness, the field of pure intelligence, simultaneously the body is losing stresses and strains, and thereby the clouds that were hindering the use of inner full creative intelligence in action, they begin to wither away.

As a result of staying clean and sober for many years and devoting myself to daily meditation and yoga, my intuitive nature has developed greatly. Having talked to many people in recovery who also have a dedicated meditation or yoga practice, I have found that they too have been able to enhance their intuition. This does not mean that they do not make mistakes but they are much more in tune with potential external pitfalls. They find it much easier to make wise choices and sound decisions.

Bathing in being

It has been said by many spiritual teachers throughout the ages that we are 'human beings', not 'human doings'. It is also true that life tends to work out much better if we learn how to 'be' before we 'do'. When we operate from a place of being, it is easier to observe any dysfunctional patterns of behaviour we might be repeating that are preventing us from leading a fulfilling and functional life. We can be much more flexible and resilient when we are anchored in our True Selves and are present as often as possible. In my view we are spiritual beings having a human experience and when we have learned to *be*, to feel our feelings gracefully and realize that our life is really a meditation, we can integrate our higher spiritual True Self with the mind and body.

Cultivating warm-heartedness

The process of self-kindness strengthens a desire to practise warm-heartedness towards our fellow human beings. As we learn to love ourselves and take care of our human needs, the wish to be charitable, kind, loving and compassionate becomes a natural way to live. As a result of gradually forgiving ourselves for our shortcomings we can view others in a new compassionate light. We can see people as human beings, with desirable characteristics and human shortcomings. Being of service to humanity and the planet becomes fulfilling because we no longer want to manipulate people for our own ends. We serve for the sake of serving. Serving others is a spiritual act. If we need or want something we can be frank and honest, while ulterior motives and fearful choices recede.

10

Make peace with yourself

Practising self-kindness

The power of self-kindness can help us to heal our chronic shame and self-loathing. In a world that is often mean-spirited and cruel, a daily practice of kindness and warm-heartedness can make all the difference. When we relearn to love ourselves and practise daily super self-care and self-kindness, the healing process can unfold. This is not easy, but it is possible. The key thing to remember when practising self-kindness is to be gentle in our approach.

Emotionally wounded addicts have harmed themselves in the most dehumanizing ways. Self-kindness is the opposite of creating self-inflicted wounds. Self-kindness is being gentle with ourselves. If we do not take care of ourselves properly it will be increasingly difficult to be authentically kind to others. When our minds and bodies are consumed with anxiety and fear, deciding to read a passage from a good recovery book, going for a walk to call on a friend in recovery or meditating is an act of self-kindness. If we are making small strides every day to improve our spiritual practice, this is self-kindness in action. For people recovering from addictive behaviour, self-kindness is truly wonderful.

Affirmations do not work unless we address our frozen grief

Many people report that repeating affirmations out loud did not work for them. They soon became bored and stopped repeating their affirmations altogether. Repeating affirmations without going through the process of properly grieving our losses and childhood trauma will be in vain. I used to repeat affirmations with little result until I started to *feel* my darkest feelings in recovery. An emotionally wounded addict can repeat an affirmation one hundred times a day for three months and still have no major breakthroughs in his consciousness. However, a person who is going through her grief work and repeating several affirmations once a day for 30 days can start to see an improvement in her sense of self-worth.

Below are some helpful affirmations that are worth reading out loud. Rather than being rigid, it is better to spontaneously read several affirmations out loud twice a week. I have used these affirmations at my workshops and mindfulness retreats. You can also write out your own affirmations. Experiment.

- 'I am worthy of love and affection.'
- 'I am deeply connected to my authentic self.'
- 'I accept myself unconditionally.'
- 'I associate with people who love me for who I really am.'
- 'I cherish and honour my inner child.'
- 'I can accept today that I will never be perfect and it is OK to make mistakes.'
- 'I no longer please other people at the expense of my mental, emotional, spiritual, physical and financial well-being.'
- 'I am OK with not knowing what is going to happen in the future.'
- 'I can make peace with any traumatic events that happened to me in childhood.'
- 'My inherent worth is based on my existence here on Earth.'
- 'I love and value myself.'
- 'I no longer put myself in dangerous situations.'
- 'I am responsible for my own well-being.'
- 'I no longer wish to control how other people think and behave.'
- 'I no longer feel guilty for standing up for myself.'
- 'It is OK for me to feel angry.'
- 'It is OK for me to feel sad.'
- 'I can have fun and enjoy myself without feeling guilty.'
- 'I no longer crave the approval of my fellows.'
- 'I am a human being.'

- 'I am not above or below any other human being.'
- 'I can be successful if I learn to let go of control.'
- 'It is OK to be successful – I no longer need to feel guilty or ashamed about this.'
- 'Peace is always realized within me.'
- 'Money is an essential tool to expand my life.'
- 'Money is a reflection of services rendered.'
- 'Prosperity is a good thing.'
- 'I enjoy being positively visible and serving my fellow human beings.'
- 'I am a beautiful and intelligent human being.'
- 'I can accept with grace that my body is ageing.'
- 'I accept that no one can fix or rescue me.'
- 'I no longer allow others to violate my emotional boundaries.'
- 'I no longer need to compare myself to others.'

Letting go of perfectionism

In her book *Your Messy Brilliance* (2017), Kelly McNelis writes, 'Our society is obsessed with the idea of perfection. Whether we're looking at the carefully scripted speeches of politicians or the airbrushed and immaculately coiffed images of Hollywood actors, we live in a culture in which images of what we have defined as "perfect" are everywhere.'

While excellence is a wonderful ideal, perfection is a dysfunctional belief system. Many people openly admit that they are perfectionists, which is really an unconscious cry for help. Being a perfectionist is really stating that whatever we attempt to do will never be good enough. This is due to a mistaken belief that we are flawed and unlovable. Perfectionism is usually the by-product of being brought up in a rigid family system that allows no room for error. To make a mistake in a perfectionist family system is a grave violation of an unspoken rule of the dysfunctional family. The notion of being human is unacceptable. To be human leaves a person open to being ridiculed or shamed and, in some cases, to receive verbal and physical violence.

For those brought up in the perfectionist, dysfunctional family system, the constant demand to be 'flawless' creates anxiety, depression, addictive behaviour and self-loathing. Even when a family member has accomplished something outstanding, it still is not good enough within the family system or it can be mocked. The person who achieves the outstanding objective also feels that he or she is still not good enough. The perfection that we demand of ourselves is part of a deeper unrest in our consciousness. It tends to be another survival trait to mask the hurt we carry inside.

When we are able to observe and notice our tendencies to demand perfection from ourselves, we can slow down our reactive patterns and stop acting them out. Discussing perfectionism with a fellow in recovery or in a support group can pave the way for healing. When we make a conscious effort to let go of perfectionism, uncomfortable emotions will come up; however, this is part of the process. Toxic guilt and shame tend to be the driving emotions behind perfectionism. As we grieve the pain behind our compulsion to be perfect, we can take more risks in our lives, allow room for error, be spontaneous and enhance our creativity. We can transcend our rigid belief system and reduce stress, dealing with pressure in a more productive way.

Generally speaking, shame-based addicts often have unrealistically high expectations of themselves and others. This makes it almost impossible to practise self-kindness. We have to let go of demanding perfection if we are going to recover and heal.

Self-compassion and self-forgiveness

Consciously practising self-compassion is very therapeutic. As we feel our grief, we can choose to have compassion for ourselves. When we reflect on our younger selves and the unfortunate choices we made, we can direct compassion and kindness inwards. We can, as a matter of fact, gradually forgive ourselves. We can forgive ourselves for neglecting self-care and associating with people who did not have our best interests at heart. We can forgive ourselves for making mistakes that cost us relationships and money. Forgiveness directed inwards can help us to be at peace with ourselves. We can accept the past and choose to be different in the present moment.

In the early stages of practising self-compassion, toxic guilt and shame might come into play. The toxic guilt and shame we feel about the harm we have done to others might appear, causing us to question whether we deserve to be compassionate towards ourselves. We might even question whether we deserve a peaceful and abundant life. We might subconsciously affirm to ourselves by saying, 'My punishment for my actions is to be unhappy and guilty, to struggle for the rest of my life – I can't forgive myself.' If we are not mindful of this excessive guilt, it can cause us to think that we need to punish ourselves repeatedly. Consequently, we might reject opportunities to thrive and prosper. We might dismiss our talents and skills, feeling bitterly torn between wanting to be positively visible and retreating into isolation. If we do not forgive ourselves through meditation, recovery and fellowship, we might never truly be free.

Mothers in particular carry enormous guilt when they come into recovery and observe that their children are living unhappy lives, which may have resulted from addictive behaviour passed down the generations. This can make it very difficult for a mother or father attempting to practise self-forgiveness. The best thing a parent can do for his or her offspring is practise super self-care. This is the only way through the pain.

There are some things we have done that we can never 'mend' or 'change', which can be very hard to accept. We can spend years wishing that we had not behaved in such an unfortunate way. This can cause very deep emotional blockages in our consciousness, which can freeze our efforts to heal and thrive.

Before coming into recovery (and sometimes even in recovery), many of us have sought refuge in destructive environments with emotionally toxic people. We were attracted to extreme behaviours and rejected the company of people who appeared to be content and calm because we felt 'less than' around them. I sought refuge in crack houses in affluent neighbourhoods because that way I felt (falsely or not) part of a group. Many of the men and women who used to drink and use substances in these houses had had privileged upbringings; nevertheless they were drug addicts and wanted to be around others who knew what it was like to need to be intoxicated all the time. I had to revisit the chronic shame around my past in this area of my life and forgive myself.

I can remember when I started to consciously practise self-kindness and self-forgiveness in recovery. I was overwhelmed by toxic guilt. It felt selfish to be directing kindness inwards. I can still be haunted by regrettable memories, but I have much more self-acceptance than I did before I began processing my frozen pain. The reality is that if we cannot be kind to ourselves, recovery is not possible.

Focus on character building rather than trying to control everything

Seeing that we cannot control outcomes and other people, it makes sense to focus on what we can control and shape. We can unreservedly control and shape our character and attitude. If we indulge in cruel gossip or are brash or entrenched in egotism, we can with willingness and a conscious discipline change our behaviour. For example, in my teens and early twenties one of my shortcomings was arrogance. It was a characteristic that did not serve me well in recovery. As an adult in recovery, I want to be authentic and truthful whenever possible, so I have consciously dropped this undesirable behaviour over the years.

It is much better to focus on who you wish to be as a person rather than trying to control others. We can be inspired by how other people carry themselves in everyday life without losing our own sense of uniqueness. For instance, several years ago I wrote a list of people who impressed me. This list had nothing to do with their status or wealth. I focused on what they were like as people. They were kind, generous, spoke frankly and honestly, they were gracious and warm. I wanted to improve in these areas and so I made a decision to learn from the men and women on my list. Since writing that list, I have improved. It might be worth thinking about the qualities you admire in other people and see if you can make a conscious daily effort to integrate those qualities into your own character. That is something you do have control over.

Asserting emotional boundaries

It takes courage to assert new boundaries, especially when people have been accustomed to you having very few boundaries – if any at all. The fear of conflict can be terrifying for many emotionally wounded people, especially when they are suffering from complex PTSD and trauma (some, however, use conflict as an internal drug to jolt them into a sense of aliveness). By and large, people who are afraid of asserting boundaries are afraid of being shamed, losing control or being physically punished. Usually there is stored trauma in the body, which their conscious mind cannot connect with. Many emotionally wounded people freeze or flee when conflict is on the horizon.

If we are still people pleasing, setting boundaries is practically impossible. If we are rageful and fly off the handle on a regular basis it will also be difficult to assert boundaries in a non-violent way. Creating new boundaries is a process. We get better at it the more we practise and pay attention to our inner moral compass.

A woman who comes into recovery as a result of drug addiction might find that now she is clean she can no longer handle being 'managed' by her husband. The more her husband attempts to control her, the more resentment builds up inside her until one day she explodes with incandescent rage. Her husband is taken aback in disbelief; she affirms that she doesn't need to be told what to do any more. It takes time for the couple to adjust because she has been a victim for most of their 25-year marriage and the husband a 'rescuer'. The woman often has to remind her husband to stop being controlling. This leads to arguments, but she feels empowered every time she stands up for herself. She needs to continue working on this, but the more she practises, the easier it becomes.

Creating new boundaries will enhance your self-worth and self-respect. The more boundaries you create and honour, the more empowered you feel. The more empowered you feel, the more life expands. It is much easier to create and honour boundaries to protect ourselves once we have reconnected with the inner child. When we feel that we have a duty and an obligation to protect our inner child (our spirit), new power and courage flows through us.

A healthy boundary could look like asking your co-worker not to smoke near you or asking your friend to arrive on time rather than always keeping you waiting. There are all sorts of boundaries we can practise in recovery. Sometimes we will have to adjust certain boundaries as we go along; nonetheless we will find that some boundaries are non-negotiable. Rather than being rigid, experiment and see how you get on. The more you practise this, the easier it gets.

It is a misapprehension that we can give our power away to other people. It is impossible to hand it over. We can, however, neglect to demonstrate healthy and strong boundaries in everyday life. When we do not honour our boundaries it might feel as if we have given our power away; nevertheless this feeling is really a confirmation that we have not exercised a boundary.

The twelve-step programme of recovery

When a recovering alcoholic, Bill Wilson, met an untreated alcoholic, Dr Bob Smith, on 10 June 1935 for the purpose of sharing his experience of staying sober, the seed had been planted for saving the lives of tens of millions of addicts over seven decades. This important meeting of two alcohol addicts sharing their experiences, strength and hope with one another was the origin of Alcoholics Anonymous. The twelve-step recovery model has helped millions of people worldwide since the 1940s to recover from substance and process addictions. The twelve-step programme was initially developed in the early years of Alcoholics Anonymous. As a result of its long-lasting effectiveness, other recovery fellowships have since adopted the twelve-step model.*

---

* By the late 1940s it had become undeniable that the twelve-step model worked. Consequently, three large twelve-step fellowships formed in the 1950s: Al-Anon (1951), Narcotics Anonymous (1953) and Gamblers Anonymous (1957). Since the 1950s, dozens of twelve-step fellowships have emerged, addressing all sorts of addictive and compulsive behaviours.

The twelve-step model is a fellowship that provides a sense of belonging and human companionship, and it has a spiritual component too. One of the main reasons twelve-step communities are so effective is that they have a non-shaming tone, which encourages people to come out of hiding and talk. Addiction thrives in secrecy and denial, so when a man walks into a twelve-step group and says, 'My name is Tony and I am an addict', he has started the process of healing his shame, excessive guilt and fear of rejection. The secrecy around the addiction has begun to subside.

Twelve-step fellowships have been proven to minimize isolation and enhance a sense of belonging. The twelve-step programme itself consists of self-acceptance, reconnecting with one's spiritual (non-religious) nature, gentle self-appraisals, making amends to oneself and others and being of maximum service to others. All twelve-step recovery fellowships and programmes are rooted in a personal spiritual practice rather than a particular religious affiliation. Atheists, agnostics and those who follow a particular religion come together in a spirit of recovery during a twelve-step meeting.

The gift of fellowship

In 2017, I was invited to lead a mindfulness workshop and guide a live meditation on Mingus Mountain, Arizona, to over 100 men and women at a recovery retreat. On the eve of my workshop, I had the opportunity to join in a men's twelve-step meeting, which took place by the campfire in Prescott National Park Forest, with at least 40 men recovering from childhood grief and trauma. The meeting grounded us in what was a large retreat with many unfamiliar faces. I was the only mixed-race Brit, surrounded by mostly white middle-class American men (baby boomers and Generation X), yet our common bond of validating each other's wounds in recovery utterly transcended any differences of nationality, race and heritage. We shared our pain and hope in a non-shaming environment, listening and allowing every man to have his say without interruption. At the end of the meeting we stood up in a large circle and recited the serenity prayer:

> God grant me the serenity to accept the people I cannot change, the courage to change the one I can, and the wisdom to know that one is me.

After the meeting closed, I felt that I belonged and I was enthusiastic about the retreat, even though I was thousands of miles away from England.

Meeting up regularly for a cup of tea or coffee with fellow travellers in recovery has served me well over the years. I have had major breakthroughs sitting in a coffee shop and sharing what's on my mind with a handful of recovery friends. Sometimes a brief meeting for coffee before or after a support group can be as helpful as participating in the group itself.

Similarly, making regular outreach calls to my fellows in recovery has been incredibly helpful in minimizing isolation and building communication skills. It took me several years to feel comfortable calling up my peers in recovery for all sorts of reasons (usually low self-worth). I would convince myself that I was 'bothering them', even though they had given me their phone number and made it perfectly clear that it was OK to call them. Occasionally, I can still feel I am 'intruding' while making an outreach call, but the feelings of low self-worth dissolve much more speedily than hitherto.

Furthermore, when my emotional pain is too over-bearing or when I feel isolated, I pick up my phone and connect with my fellows in recovery. For instance, when I was in the middle of feeling my suppressed childhood grief and working with a fellow traveller in recovery, the emotional pain was so intense that I had to pick up the phone. It was a Sunday evening and I had just attended a support group. My fellow in recovery was going through a similar emotional episode and so our conversation was well worth the phone call. We did not comment on what we shared but conversely, we listened carefully to each other and talked about our own experience.

A phone call for the purpose of recovery can add great value in one's personal life. In most twelve-step fellowships, the telephone is encouraged as a vital recovery tool.

A gentle reflection

To gain more awareness regarding self-care, try answering the following questions. If you notice that you need to improve in a particular area, that is OK. This reflection is created to support you. It is probably a good idea to talk your answers through with a trusted friend in recovery or a professional.

- Do you neglect your well-being so that you can support other people's needs?
- Do you feel you are being selfish unless you are burning yourself out to serve loved ones, friends and work colleagues?
- Do you feel guilty and unlovable if you honour your needs and wants?
- Do you find that you say 'yes' to things when you actually mean 'no'?
- Do you feel a compulsive need to be liked and approved of?
- Do you feel guilty if you say 'no' when people ask for your time, energy and/or money?
- Do you feel that duty comes above personal well-being?

A guided loving-kindness meditation

A metta (loving-kindness) meditation is a wonderful meditation that enhances self-acceptance and compassion towards our fellow human beings. The realization behind loving-kindness meditation is that when we practise self-compassion and self-care, we can extend our warmth and love to others authentically. This is often one of the most difficult meditations for people to participate in, because loving-kindness meditation begins with the individual accepting self-compassion. Nevertheless, with gentle persistence the practice becomes familiar and the idea of loving oneself is slowly integrated. Record the scripted meditation below and play it back to yourself. Sit with the emotions you feel after listening to the recording. If you feel you need to write down the emotions that came up during the meditation, then do so.

A guided loving-kindness meditation

Close your eyes.

Observe how you are breathing effortlessly in the present moment. Notice the life breath flow within and through you. Feel the life breath sustain and heal you. Notice every inhale breath and every exhale breath. Continue to watch the breath.

Pause recording for 30 seconds.

Take a deep breath. Notice how your body is breathing automatically. Feel the breath gently enter and leave your body. Feel how your chest and tummy rise as you breathe effortlessly in the present moment. Continue observing and feeling the breath enter and leave your body.

Pause recording for 30 seconds.

Whenever your mind distracts you with thoughts, memories and mental monologues, come back to your breathing. The breath is your anchor. Come back to the nowness of life. Sense the aliveness in the body. Appreciate the subtleness of the breath.

Pause recording for 30 seconds.

Take another deep breath. Now visualize yourself sitting in a comfortable chair in a beautiful garden. It is a warm and sunny day. See yourself relaxed and appreciating the sunshine warming the back of your neck. Now repeat the following words: 'I love you. I love and accept you no matter what. I wish you warm-heartedness and love. I wish you health, happiness, prosperity and abundance. Whenever you feel uncertain or afraid, rest assured I am here for you. I do not expect perfection from you any longer. You are a human being and that is enough.'

Pause recording for 20 seconds.

Take another deep breath. Now visualize your loved ones and friends. See them all together in a sacred space. Wish them health, happiness, prosperity and abundance.

Pause recording for 20 seconds.

Breathe deeply for a moment. Now extend your loving-kindness to your fellow human beings in your village, town, city and/or region. Visualize your neighbourhood. Wish all life to heal and prosper. Wish your fellow human beings health, happiness, prosperity and abundance.

Pause recording for 20 seconds.

Take several deep breaths. Now extend your loving-kindness and warm-heartedness to those who have harmed you. Wish them good health, compassion, prosperity and good fortune.

Pause recording for 20 seconds.

Take another deep breath. Now visualize the planet and imagine the billions of people all over the world. See the billions of other life forms (perhaps a starfish, a lion or a dolphin) and the Earth itself. Now wish all life on Earth to thrive and prosper. Wish the ecosystem and the economic system, and the planet itself, the very best.

Pause recording for 20 seconds.

Now take several deep breaths and open your eyes.

References

Chopra, Deepak (2014) 'God is pure awareness'. Available on YouTube at: www.youtube.com/watch?v=3xp2PylIIjo

Chopra, Deepak and Tanzi, Rudolph (2013) *Super Brain: Unleashing the explosive power of your mind to maximize health, happiness, and spiritual well-being.* London: Rider.

Dines, Christopher (2013) *Manifest Your Bliss: A spiritual guide to inner peace.* London: La Petite Fleur Publishing.

— (2017) 'Recovering from the effects of growing up in an alcoholic home'. Available online at: www.huffingtonpost.co.uk/christopher-dines/recovering-from-the-effec_b_13121788.html

Dines, Christopher and Mariposa, Dr Barbara (2016) *The Kindness Habit: Transforming our relationship to addictive behaviours.* London: Riverbank Books. Pp. 9 and 46.

Godman, David (ed.) (n.d.) 'Self-atma: The teachings of Sri Ramana Maharshi'. Available online at: www.adishakti.org/_/self-atma_the_teachings_of_sri_ramana_maharshi_part_one.htm

Jain, Dr Shamini and Chopra, Dr Deepak (2015) 'Biofield science and the future of healing'. Available on YouTube at: www.youtube.com/watch?v=If6kcD8WiEg&app=desktop

McGreevey, Sue (2011) 'Eight weeks to a better brain', *The Harvard Gazette*, 21 January. Available online at: http://news.harvard.edu/gazette/story/2011/01/eight-weeks-to-a-better-brain

McNelis, Kelly (2017) *Your Messy Brilliance: 7 tools for the imperfectly perfect woman.* Acton, Ontario: Enrealment Press. P. 35.

Maharishi Mahesh Yogi (1972) Lecture at Jones Hall, Houston, TX. Available online, quoted by Mario Osatti in 'Human suffering and stress: How can transcendental meditation help?', *TM BLog*, 16 February, 2013, at: www.tm.org/blog/maharishi/basic-cause-of-human-suffering

Paul, Marla (2016) 'Rhythm of breathing affects memory and fear', *Northwestern Now*, 7 December. Available online at: https://news.northwestern.edu/stories/2016/12/rhythm-of-breathing-affects-memory-and-fear

Sex and Love Addicts Anonymous (n.d.) 'Does anorexia tie in to your sex and love addiction?' Available online at: https://slaafws.org/anorexia-questionaire

Underearners Anonymous (2017) 'About Underearners Anonymous'. See website: www.underearnersanonymous.org

University of Cambridge (2014) 'Brain activity in sex addiction mirrors that of drug addiction', 11 July. Available online at: www.cam.ac.uk/research/news/brain-activity-in-sex-addiction-mirrors-that-of-drug-addiction

Wilson, Bill (1958) 'The next frontier: Emotional sobriety', Grapevine Article 22, Silkworth.net. Available online at: http://silkworth.net/aahistory/emotionalsobriety.html

Wilson, Gary (2015) *Your Brain on Porn: Internet pornography and the emerging science of addiction*. Taipei: Commonwealth Publishing.